Contents

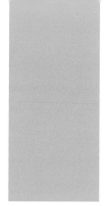

KU-308-397

Orthopaedic Diagnosis and Management

A Guide to the Care of Orthopaedic Patients
Second Edition

Boyd S. Goldie BSc (Hons) FRCS

Consultant Orthopaedic Surgeon,
Whipps Cross Hospital, London, UK

I S I S
MEDICAL
MEDIA

Oxford

© 1998 by Isis Medical Media Ltd.
59 St Aldates, Oxford OX1 1ST, UK

First edition (published by Blackwell Scientific Publications, Oxford) 1992
Second edition 1998

British Library Cataloguing in Publication Data.
A catalogue record for this title is available from
the British Library.

ISBN 1 899066 90 X

Goldie, B. S. (Boyd)
Orthopaedic diagnosis and management (2nd Edition)
Boyd S. Goldie

Always refer to the manufacturer's Prescribing Information before prescribing
drugs cited in this book.

Typeset by
Expo Holdings Sdn Bhd., Malaysia

Printed and bound by
Book Print, S.L., Spain

Distributed in the USA by
Mosby-Year Book, Inc, 11830 Westline Industrial Drive
St Louis MO63145, USA

Distributed in the rest of the world by
Oxford University Press, Saxon Way West, Corby
Northamptonshire NN18 9ES, UK

Preface to 1st edition

The stimulus for the production of this book came from the repetitive nature of House Officers' questions about the common orthopaedic conditions and operations. Having used the excellent *Surgical Diagnosis and Management* by David Dunn and Nigel Rawlinson, I decided that the same format should be continued in this book.

The book is designed to be carried in the white coat pocket for rapid reference. The aim of the book is to answer the questions commonly asked by students and junior doctors such as: What is the condition? How do you diagnose the condition? How do you decide when surgery is required? What does the operation entail? What is the management before and after the operation? What complications do you need to know about in order to obtain a proper consent?

In addition, I have tried to give answers to the common questions asked by patients of their doctors: How long will I be in hospital? How long does the operation take? Will I be in a plaster afterwards? When will I be able to go back to work?

I have given what are generally acceptable answers to these questions and I am grateful to the Consultants who have carefully checked the text.

This book aims to give guidance only about orthopaedic surgery. For newly qualified House Officers whose orthopaedic job is their first, I strongly recommend that they read the introductory chapters 'The daily management of patients in surgical wards' and 'Prescriptions and other tasks' in *Surgical Diagnosis and Management*, since these apply as much to the orthopaedic patient as the general surgical patient.

I hope that this book will make the task of being a junior orthopaedic doctor more fulfilling and less stressful.

Boyd S. Goldie
The Royal London Hospital

Preface to 2nd edition

When I originally thought of writing the first edition of this book I was a Senior Registrar and my aim was to make the life of the Junior Doctor easier. I wished to provide answers to the questions commonly asked of senior doctors by their juniors and of doctors by their patients. I seemed to have achieved this initial aim and the first edition sold out.

In the intervening years there has been an increasing emphasis on providing information for the patient to improve the quality of their care. There is also a greater emphasis on risk management whereby one tries to identify problems in advance so as to avoid them. By providing the information within this book to the members of the orthopaedic team, inefficiency and complications can be reduced.

I have expanded the book to include 12 new chapters. All the other chapters have been updated and revised. This edition now includes a few line drawings. In spite of this expansion, the book is still designed to fit into the pocket of a white coat.

My hope is that all personnel involved in the care of orthopaedic patients will continue to find this book a useful source of information that is often not available in standard texts. I am trying to ensure that both the patient and the medical team are fully informed about the nature of a problem, what the treatment involves and the risks and hazards of that treatment. By doing this, I wish to improve patients' satisfaction and the carers' job fulfilment.

Boyd S. Goldie
Whipps Cross Hospital

Acknowledgements

I wish to thank Mr David Dunn for allowing me to continue to use the format that he originated for *Surgical Diagnosis and Management*. My thanks also go to John Harrison for encouraging me to write a second edition of this book.

My main debt of gratitude is owed to my wife who yet again has put up with my absences and yet again has acted as proofreader.

B.S.G.

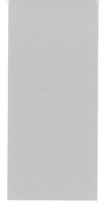

The layout of this book

The first chapters present overviews on the management of orthopaedic patients, fractures, osteoarthritis, rheumatoid arthritis and common complications. After that the chapters are arranged anatomically. Each subject is presented using some or all of the headings described below.

The condition

This is a thumbnail sketch of the condition, with some reference to incidence and aetiology.

Making the diagnosis

The patient

Although there are always exceptions, it is often possible to describe the typical patient who is suffering from a particular condition. Remember that I am giving a pattern for ease of identification but that there are always patients who are atypical.

The history

As in all clinical medicine, the history is the key to most diagnoses. A complete history, including the patient's general health and social history, must not be skimped upon. This applies even when the radiograph that may have been viewed before seeing the patient shows an obvious disorder. I give certain key points for each condition that will help to keep the history concise.

On examination

I have outlined the most relevant points in the examination. However, certain signs are difficult to describe and are best demonstrated. You should never hesitate to ask your seniors to demonstrate an examination that is unfamiliar to you.

Radiographs

The term 'X-ray' is avoided since it is medical slang. An X-ray beam is a beam of electromagnetic radiation and is invisible. What we look at is the developed film after it has been exposed to the X-rays. This is more properly called a radiograph. Although this may seem pedantic, many surgeons will delight in the opportunity to correct students and junior doctors.

Preoperative management

Investigations

It is assumed that you will order the appropriate investigations for the patient's age, medical history and race. I mention only additional investigations that are relevant to the orthopaedic condition.

Common associated injuries

Patients who have suffered trauma often have injuries that are not immediately apparent at presentation. Always try to consider the possibility that there is another injury. Do not home in on the obvious. Remember that one-third of inpatients with a fracture have a second injury diagnosed after admission.

Preparation for surgery

Treatment

I give the treatment choices for the diagnosis. This includes conservative treatment such as physiotherapy and outpatient treatment such as local steroid injections.

Indications for surgery

Certain symptoms and signs must be present as indications for specific operations. If they are absent, the surgery for which the patient has been admitted may be inappropriate and even counterproductive. This is very important in elective patients who may have been on the waiting list for months (or years) before being admitted. During the time between being placed on the waiting list and admission, the patient may completely recover or deteriorate so much that a different operation is indicated. If your history and examination makes you question the proposed treatment plan, do not hesitate to inform the surgeon.

Operation

The aim of the description of the procedure is to allow you, the house officer, to understand what is to be done and thus achieve a consent where both doctor and patient are informed!

Codes

These are only meant to be a guide. There is a wide variation in the practice of different surgeons and I suggest that you amend the codes as necessary.

- GA/LA. GA, general anaesthetic; LA, local anaesthetic, includes spinal, epidural and intravenous regional anaesthetics.
- Blood. This is a guide as to how much blood to cross match, and not to the average blood loss. Many hospitals have policies as to how much blood to make available for common operations, and it is wise to check on this. However, it is the surgical team's responsibility to ensure that an adequate quantity of blood is cross matched, whatever the local guidelines.
- Antibiotics. The typical prophylaxis for orthopaedic procedures is three doses of an intravenous antibiotic, with the first dose given on induction of anaesthesia. The most commonly prescribed antibiotic for prophylaxis is a cephalosporin. Regimes, however, vary from surgeon to surgeon. If you are in any doubt, ask.
- Time. The time given is only a very rough guide to the length of operation. It is obviously very variable, but it is given because many patients ask how long their operation will take. You should always explain that this is only the length of the operation itself. The time between leaving the ward and arriving back is much longer.
- Drains. Most orthopaedic surgeons do not suture in the drains. Generally, most drainage occurs in the first 24 hours postoperatively. Leaving the drains in longer increases the risk of infection and so drains are usually removed 24 hours after surgery.

- Plaster. Most limbs swell following surgery. If plaster immobilization is required, we either apply a well-padded back-slab or a full plaster that is immediately split. If a patient has severe postoperative pain, the plaster and dressings must be split *down to the skin*.
- Postoperative radiograph. Operations on bones usually require a check radiograph, whereas soft tissue operations do not. The appropriate views have been suggested. The ideal time for taking the radiograph is dealt with under 'Postoperative care' (see below).
- Stay. Again, only a rough guide to the length of stay postoperatively is given. This is probably the most common question to be asked by patients.
- Follow-up. If the patient needs to have sutures removed following their operation, they need to be seen in the clinic about 10 days after their operation. If the patient has a fracture that may move, they will need to be seen for a check radiograph 1 week after discharge. If the above does not apply, patients are usually seen 6 weeks following surgery. Always ask the surgeon about the time of the follow-up appointment if you are in any doubt.
- Off work. The length of time that a patient will be off work depends on their operation and the nature of their work. Remember that many patients with sedentary occupations, who have surgery to their lower limbs, are often off work purely due to being unable to use public transport.

Operative requirements

Many orthopaedic operations involve specialized equipment. However, the theatre staff may not always know from the title of the operation on the theatre list, what equipment is required. Therefore, the theatre staff should be told in advance what is likely to be needed. It is also good practice to write what equipment is needed on the operating list.

Postoperative care

Management

Much of the guidance relates to the mobilization of the patient. The surgeon should always state what he wants, so that you, the patient, the nursing staff and the physiotherapists all work to the same plan.

Complications

The complications listed are those associated with that particular operation. For a full, informed consent, you should explain the orthopaedic risks and also the risks of the anaesthetic and blood transfusion. If you write the headings of the complications that you discuss with the patient on the consent form as you discuss them, you will be able to assure a court with greater conviction that they were indeed mentioned!

Daily management of patients in orthopaedic wards

Patient records

It is vital that every entry is legible, relevant and clearly signed. Every history sheet must have the patient's name and hospital number on it. This is because pages often come adrift from the notes and it can be difficult to identify loose bits of paper. In addition, claims for negligence are difficult to refute when the notes are poor or absent.

Pre-admission clinic

Most departments run a pre-admission clinic for patients undergoing elective surgery. You should review the notes of the patients in advance. Write out the forms for blood tests, urine tests, ECG and radiographs before the clinic starts, to save time later. You may want to send some of the patients for their tests while you see the first patients.

Ideally the clinic should be arranged so the Consultant can see the patients as well. This is especially important now that many operations are performed as day cases or overnight stays. The surgeon cannot see these patients on a ward round the day before surgery and must see the patients at some point before their arrival in the anaesthetic room.

Review the results of the tests that you order as soon as they are available. One of the main purposes of a pre-admission clinic is to avoid patient's operations being cancelled once they have been admitted. If a test shows that the patient is unfit for surgery, the operation can be postponed and another patient brought in to fill the space.

If a patient does not attend the pre-admission clinic, tell your consultant so that the list can be reorganized and another patient sent for.

Patient information leaflets

Many departments have information leaflets for patients. The ideal leaflet should contain information about all aspects of the patient's treatment. The nature of the problem should be explained in an understandable manner. The risks and hazards of the treatment should be included. If you have access to leaflets you should give them out to every patient. The aim is for the patient to be fully informed. This will hopefully avoid patient dissatisfaction that commonly results from poor communication.

Information leaflets that complement this book are available from Scalpel Information Systems, 12 Staindrop Road, Darlington, Co Durham DL3 9AE.

Preoperative check

You should make a check list in the notes with a tick next to each item to show that the task has been performed. You should write the results of key blood test in the notes. This list should include the following:

Laboratory tests
Not all patients need the following tests. Refer to *Surgical Diagnosis and Management* (Dunn and Rawlinson; Blackwell Scientific Publications, 1991) for guidelines.

FBC U&E	Write out the blood results in red
CXR	Look at the radiograph yourself and write something to show that you have done so, e.g. lungs clear
ECG	Look at the ECG and make a note, e.g. sinus rhythm
Cross match	Note the amount

Mark the site and side of operation

To avoid operating on the incorrect side, you must mark the operation site with an arrow using an indelible marker. You must mark the site before the patient receives their premedication so that you and the patient can agree that the correct side is marked.

Do not put the arrow on the site of the incision. For a total hip replacement, an arrow drawn just above the knee, pointing to the appropriate hip, is adequate. For finger and toe operations, the surgeon could potentially operate on the wrong digit. Draw an arrow, indicating the correct digit, on *both* sides of the hand or foot.

In spite of the above, it is ultimately the surgeon's responsibility to check that he is doing the correct operation on the correct patient.

Radiographs

Ensure that the radiographs are on the ward preoperatively and that they arrive in theatre with the patient. Once in theatre, put the most recent appropriate radiograph onto the screen.

Consent

The house surgeon usually obtains the consent for surgery from the patient. It is therefore your responsibility to ensure that the description of the operation is accurate, and includes the side and digit where relevant. The writing on the form must be legible, including your signature. Abbreviations must be avoided. If you have given the patient an information leaflet that explains the nature of the operation and its risks and hazards, you should note this on the consent.

Operating list

In most hospitals it is the house surgeon's responsibility to write out the operating list that is handed to the theatre secretary for typing and distribution. It is vital that the theatre list is accurate and complete for both the patients' safety and for medico-legal reasons.

- The order of the list must be decided by the surgeon. In general, children are put at the beginning of the list, as are diabetic patients. Infected or dirty cases are operated on at the end of the list.
- The exact nature of each operation must be given, stating any prosthesis or special equipment that is needed.
- Use capital letters and do not use abbreviations, even for the side to be operated upon.

- Theatres must also be informed if the patient is a potential bio-hazard, e.g. hepatitis B or AIDS.
- Make a note if the image intensifier in theatre is needed, as a copy of the list is usually sent to the X-ray department. In addition always inform the X-ray department, well in advance, if they are likely to be needed.

Tourniquet

The tourniquet is a pneumatically inflated cuff. It is commonly used in upper and lower limb operations to allow the surgeon to operate in a bloodless field. It is often the house officer's task to apply the tourniquet. The appropriate size of cuff must be chosen relative to the size of the limb. There are a selection of cuffs, from those small enough for a baby, to those large enough to go around a large adult thigh. The use of the wrong size can lead to either inadequate or excessive compression.

Wrap the area that will be under the tourniquet with a protective layer of plaster wool. Apply the tourniquet as snugly as possible and then connect it to the inflation box. Exsanguinate the limb either by using an Esmarch bandage or the Rhys Davis exsanguinator. Both require a modicum of skill and you should be shown how to use them. When the limb is exsanguinated, inflate the tourniquet to a pressure of 100 mmHg above the patient's systolic blood pressure. It is best to set the desired pressure before inflating the cuff, and then turn the switch to inflate. This rapidly inflates the cuff to the correct pressure. If the switch is turned to inflate and the pressure slowly increased, you will occlude the veins before the arteries and end up with a poor exsanguination. This leads to an irritating ooze into the wound.

When the patient is prepped you must ensure that no antiseptic gets under the tourniquet. With iodine based antiseptics, the pressure of the tourniquet on the iodine soaked wool can cause skin burns. This is most likely if the limb is to be prepped close to the tourniquet. Either wrap waterproof tape (e.g. sleek) over the distal edge of the cuff or put a U drape just distal to the tourniquet before applying the antiseptic.

The time of inflation should be noted. The tourniquet is best deflated after 1.5 hours for the upper limb, and 2 hours for the lower limb.

Operation notes

These are written immediately after each procedure by either the surgeon or the assistant. If they are written onto ordinary history sheets it is best to write in red. This makes it easy to find the operation note among the rest of the notes. Some hospitals have separate sheets for the operations notes.

In some departments, the surgeon dictates an operation note that is typed and then inserted into the notes. Since it may take several days for the typed note to reach the patient's file, it is important that a brief note is also written. You should ask the secretary to make a copy of every typed note that has your name on. Not only will this help you compile your log book, but it may be useful to refer to operative details in the future.

The information recorded in the operation note should include the following:
- Date.
- Title of the operation, e.g. cemented CPT total hip replacement.
- Surgeon.
- Assistant.
- Anaesthetist.
- Type of anaesthetic, e.g. GA, LA, Biers, axillary.
- Tourniquet time.
- Incision/approach, e.g. modified lateral to hip. This is important for postoperative mobilization in operations around the hip, as patients who have had a posterior approach are not generally allowed to sit out of bed as early as those who have had the lateral or anterolateral approach.
- Findings. The extent of the handwritten description depends upon whether or not a note is dictated for typing. A drawing of an injury or arthroscopic examination can often be helpful.
- Procedure. If an implant has been used, record the type and size. For a total hip replacement this must include the outside diameter of

the acetabulum, the head diameter, the size of the femoral component, the neck length and whether or not a cement restrictor was
used. The manufacturer's labels, with the batch number for each
component, must be attached to the notes. For a fracture, record
the type of plate and the number of screws inserted.

■ Closure. Record:
(a) the number and type of drains, e.g. 2 redivacs;
(b) the type of suture to deep layers, e.g. No. 1 Vicryl to muscle and
2/0 Vicryl to subcutaneous layers;
(c) the type and nature of skin closure, e.g. continuous subcuticular
PDS or interrupted nylon.

■ Postoperative instructions. These are the most important part of the
operation notes. These are the guides for the nursing staff and the
on-call doctor. The instructions should state what particular observations must be made, mobilization instructions, when the drains are
to be removed and how long antibiotics are to be continued.

For a routine total hip replacement they may be as follows:
(a) routine mobilization for posterior approach;
(b) drains out at 24 hours;
(c) AP pelvis on return to ward;
(d) two further doses Cefuroxime;
(e) sutures out at 10 days.

If there is a possibility that the neuro-vascular status could deteriorate, regular neuro-vascular observations must be made. It is not
sufficient to simply write 'monitor neuro-vasc obs' in the postoperative
instructions. State what observations must be made and how often.
This is especially important following operations where there is a risk of
compartment syndrome. You should write:

*Monitor foot pulses, toe sensation and pain on toe extension hourly for
12 hours, 2 hourly for the next 12 hours and then 4 hourly until 48 hours.*

There is then no doubt about what has to be observed and for how
long.

Day cases

Every patient should be seen before going home. The patient must go
home with adequate painkillers. They must have clear instructions on

what they may and may not do at home. They need an outpatient appointment. The patient ought to be given the discharge letter to pass onto their GP. This must clearly state what the patient has had done, what drugs they have been given and what the follow-up arrangements are.

Postoperative care of inpatients

At the end of the case, the house officer should write up the antibiotic prophylaxis regime on the prescription chart. It will save you time if you write out the forms for the check haemoglobin and the check radiograph while in theatre (waiting for the next case to begin!).

On the day of surgery, every postoperative patient should have a postoperative check by the duty house officer. A note must be made in the file and should include a comment about neuro-vascular function and the amount of drainage.

Subsequent postoperative notes should record whether or not the check radiographs were satisfactory, after what interval the drains were removed, the total drainage during and after surgery, and the postoperative blood results. Each entry must be dated. For ease of reference, the number of postoperative days can be noted at the start of the entry, e.g. 'POD 1' for the first postoperative day.

For any operation where the patient loses a significant amount of blood (for an adult this would be greater than 200 ml), the haemoglobin should be measured on the second postoperative day.

A check radiograph is usually required after most orthopaedic operations, except after purely soft tissue operations. In lower limb operations this radiograph is usually obtained before the patient is allowed out of bed. The optimal time to take a check radiograph varies from hospital to hospital. The ideal time (from a surgeon's point of view) is in the recovery room. This allows the surgeon to check the radiograph while the patient could potentially return to the theatre to correct any disaster. In addition, the patient while in recovery still has adequate analgesia. This means that the positioning that is required to take the radiograph is not too distressing for the patient. However, obtaining check radiographs in recovery requires considerable cooperation from the X-ray department.

In some hospitals, the patient returns to the ward via the X-ray department. This occupies a recovery nurse for an additional length of time. It may be dangerous for a patient who has undergone a major operation to be in the X-ray department away from monitoring and resuscitation equipment. For major cases (e.g. total hip replacement), it may be best to wait until the second postoperative day to take the check radiograph, as the patient may find the positioning very uncomfortable.

An entry should be made at least daily, for all postoperative patients. Even for long stay patients, an attempt should be made to see each patient and record a note daily. There is no excuse for lack of entries in the notes, and the coroner will ask for an explanation if a patient dies with inadequate notes.

Ward rounds

A note should be made for all rounds, stating whose round it was and exactly what policy decisions were made.

For consultant ward rounds there are several hints to ensure that things run smoothly.

1. Present each patient concisely, mentioning the patient's name, age, diagnosis (including the side) and length of time since either admission or operation. If you have problems remembering who has had what and when, write a list of the patients in the order that they are to be seen.

2. Organize the radiographs *before* the ward round. If the patient is due to have an operation, have the most recent relevant radiographs at the front of the packet. If the patient had a fracture treated, have the immediate preoperative and the recent postoperative radiographs to hand. There is nothing worse than watching the house officer struggle with a pile of radiographs that seem to have a mind of their own.

3. Become acquainted with the correct orientation of radiographs – if in doubt, ask.

CHAPTER 2

Fractures

The condition

A fracture is a break in continuity of a bone. There is no difference between a break and a fracture (as many patients suppose).

A fracture may be closed or open. 'Closed' means that the skin over the fracture is intact. 'Open' means that there is a wound near the fracture and there is potential communication between the fracture and the wound. A compound fracture is the same as an open fracture.

Making the diagnosis

The patient

Certain fractures occur commonly in certain patients. The main variable is age. For example, a fall onto the outstretched hand commonly results in the following:

Toddler	Greenstick fracture of the distal radius
Infant	Injury to the distal radial epiphysis
10–15 years	Fractured clavicle
Young adult	Scaphoid fracture
Middle aged, elderly	Colles' fracture

The history

The symptoms of a fracture are pain and loss of function. The intensity of the pain may vary in different patients with similar fractures. Do not be dissuaded from asking for a radiograph if the patient only has minimal pain if you otherwise think that there could be a fracture. Remember that pain may be referred. Pain in the knee for example, may be due to an injury to the hip. The loss of function associated with a fracture may be complete, e.g. being unable to weight bear with a tibial fracture. There may be only partial loss of function, such as pain on using the wrist with a scaphoid fracture.

Always ask about loss of power or abnormal sensation distal to the fracture. This may indicate a nerve or vessel injury associated with the fracture.

When taking the history, you must document when the injury occurred and in what environment (very important if it is an open fracture). Try to establish the exact mechanism of injury. Simply knowing that the patient was playing football is not enough. The attitude of the hand when falling will often predict the configuration of the fracture.

Enquire about any symptoms away from the obviously broken bone, in particular, the adjacent joints.

If the upper limb is injured, ask the patient if they are right or left-handed. Always take a social history. Treatment of the fracture may be influenced by the occupation of the patient. For example, a metacarpal fracture in the left hand of a professional violinist might need internal fixation whereas that of a psychiatrist may not! Any patient, of any age, who lives alone is severely disabled by a cast. Ensure that the patient will be able to look after themselves if they are sent home with a leg or arm in a plaster cast.

On examination

If the patient has had a high energy injury, such as a car accident or a fall from a height, examine the whole patient carefully. Although there may be an injury that is obvious, there could be other fractures that can be missed.

The following classical signs of a fracture may or may not be present:

- *Deformity.* Deformity may be gross or subtle.
- *Swelling.* Fracture of a bone is usually associated with a varying degree of soft tissue swelling. If there is massive swelling, there may also be fracture blisters. It is important that you note the presence of these blisters, as they can get infected.
- *Tenderness.* Gently examine the patient to determine the exact site of tenderness.
- *Crepitus.* You should not deliberately try to elicit this grating of the two ends of the fractured bone.

Try to examine the adjacent joints. Obviously you cannot test the range of movement of the knee with an unstable tibial fracture, but you can look for swelling, bruising and tenderness.

Note any wound or soft tissue damage. Document the size of the wound, its location and whether it seems clean or contaminated.

Check on the integrity of neuro-vascular function distal to the fracture. Essentially this means feeling the pulses, checking sensation and asking the patient to move their fingers or toes.

Radiographs
Radiographs must be in two planes and include the whole bone with the adjacent joints.

When describing a fracture on a radiograph (often by telephone) try to answer the following questions:

1. Which bone?
2. Which side, left or right?
3. What part of the bone? For long bones, consider the bones in thirds, e.g. the fracture may be in the distal third or at the junction of the middle and distal thirds.
4. Is the fracture intra-articular? If the fracture is near a joint, does it extend into that joint?
5. Is the adjacent joint intact? Or is there a subluxation or dislocation?
6. What is the configuration of the fracture? Are there two or three major fragments, or is the fracture comminuted? Is the fracture transverse, oblique, spiral? Is there a butterfly fragment? If the fracture is due to the pull of a tendon, the fragment may look as if it has been avulsed.
7. How displaced is the fracture? Displacement must be described for each of the two planes of the radiographs. Displacement may be:

   (a) sideways shift or translocation – if so estimate the amount in relation to the width of the bone (e.g. shifted by 50% of the width of the cortex on the AP view);

   (b) angulation – describe the distal fragment in relation to the proximal;

   (c) torsion – this is usually more obvious clinically, but an AP view of the knee with a lateral view of the ankle on a single radiograph implies considerable rotation.

Preoperative management

Investigations
Some fractures need more than just plain radiographs. Tomograms or CT scans are commonly required for spinal fractures and fractures involving a joint.

Common associated injuries
Nerves, vessels and tendons can all be injured.

Treatment

Fractures that are displaced may need to be reduced. The reasons for reducing a fracture include:

- Improving the function after the fracture has united.
- Increasing the chance of union of the fracture.
- Minimizing the risk of late arthritis if the fracture is adjacent to a joint or intra-articular.
- Cosmesis.

The fracture can be reduced by manipulation, traction or open reduction. Once reduced, the position needs to be maintained. There are several ways of achieving this.

Anatomy of fracture   Some fractures are inherently stable and do not require additional stabilization.

Plaster cast   The position may be held by a cast that includes both the adjacent joints if the fracture is in the middle of a bone, or only the nearby joint if the fracture is at the end of a bone.

External fixator   If the fracture is open, the position is usually held with an external fixator. This method allows wound management while holding the fracture reduced (see Chapter 3). External fixators may be used for closed fractures if the comminution precludes successful treatment by either an external cast or internal fixation.

Traction   Fractures may be reduced and/or held by traction. Traction may be by skin traction, where adhesive tape is stuck to the limb distal to the fracture and weights applied. The amount of weight that can be applied through skin traction is limited to 2.27 kg (5 lbs). More weight than this can result in skin damage. Skin traction is used on children as the definitive form of traction for hip and femoral fractures. In the elderly, skin traction is applied as a means of temporary immobilization in patients with a femoral neck fracture. Skeletal traction is applied via a pin inserted into or through the bone. The advantages of skeletal traction over skin traction are that the weight that can be applied is much greater and traction can be continued for longer.

Internal fixation Fractures can be internally fixed after reduction by either plates and screws applied to the bone, or by devices that pass down inside the medullary cavity of a long bone. The advantages of successful internal fixation are twofold. First, accurate reduction of intra-articular fractures minimizes the risk of degenerative change in the joint. Secondly, a strong stable fixation allows early return of function of the limb. The disadvantages of internal fixation are the risk of infection and of not achieving the aim of a stable strong reduction that goes on to solid union.

Applying a plaster

Many hospitals employ a plaster technician who applies plasters for the casualty department and the fracture clinic. A technician is not usually present at night or in theatre and the house officer is often required to apply back-slabs and full plasters. You must take every opportunity to learn how to apply a plaster from the plaster technician, the registrars and the consultants.

There are several tips to make your plastering easier:

1. If the limb has not been operated upon, you can put a Tubinet bandage on the limb first. Make sure that it is not too tight and do not use Tubigrip. Apply plaster wool smoothly over the Tubinet. Remember that any bumps may become areas of high pressure and result in pressure sores under the plaster.

2. Plaster of Paris sets by an exothermic reaction and thus gets hot. If hot water is used to wet the plaster, the already hot water is further heated and it is possible to burn the patient. Therefore, use cool or tepid water. This also slows the rate at which the plaster sets and gives you more time to apply the cast.

3. Remember that any indentation that is made in the plaster as it is setting will remain and can cause a pressure sore. When holding a limb

that is being plastered, try to hold it by parts that are not being included in the plaster, e.g. the toes and above the knee for a below-knee plaster. If this is not possible, support the limb with the palm of the hand rather than the fingertips. Always hold the limb in the position in which it is to remain. In other words do not bend an elbow or a knee after applying the wool or the plaster, as the wool and plaster may cause neuro-vascular compression.

4. If the plaster is being applied to an acutely injured limb or one that has been operated upon, there is a risk of swelling. In this case, either put on a back-slab, or a full plaster that is split longitudinally.

5. Fibreglass casting material should not be used by the inexperienced, as it is difficult to use and quite unforgiving.

6. Learn how to use the plaster saw and the implements for removing a plaster. The blade of the plaster saw does not rotate, but oscillates. In theory if the blade touches the skin, it will not cut it. Always explain this to patients, who are naturally apprehensive when first confronted with the plaster saw. Remember not to drag the blade down the plaster but to use repeated downward cuts. Try to use different parts of the blade, as it can become quite hot.

Removal of K-wires and traction pins

It is often the house officer's task to remove K-wires and traction pins from patients on the ward. Both wires and pins can be removed without local anaesthetic from adults. This should be done in a clean area, such as the treatment room. It is often best to give the patient an analgesic prior to the pin extraction. Tell the nursing staff when you intend to remove the pin, so that they can give the analgesic in good time.

For a K-wire that is protruding through the skin, you will need a large needle holder or some pliers, gloves, antiseptic solution and a small dressing pack containing gauze, forceps and a small receptacle. Look at the position of the pin on the radiograph and work out in which direction you have to pull. Thoroughly clean the pin and the surrounding skin. Firmly grasp the pin, twist it and pull hard. If the wire does not come out easily, try one more time to remove it before asking the advice of a more senior person.

Femoral and tibial traction pins pass completely through the leg and it is important not to draw infection into the bone when the pin is removed. You need a dressing pack, antiseptic solution, gloves and a 'Jacob's chuck and key'. Look at the radiograph to see if the pin has threads in the middle. Alternatively, look in the notes to see if the pin is a Denham pin, which is threaded, or a Steinmann pin, which is smooth. Thoroughly clean the pin, removing all congealed blood and debris from the side of the pin that is to pass through the bone. Remove the pin using the Jacob's chuck and put dressings over the holes. If the holes ooze a lot, wrap the limb with plaster wool and a crêpe bandage.

CHAPTER 3

Open fractures

The condition

An open (compound) fracture is a fracture associated with a break in the overlying skin. The break in the skin may be due to the end of the broken bone coming out through the skin. This is referred to as compound from within. Alternatively the skin may be broken by the external impact that broke the underlying bone. Open fractures have a great risk of becoming infected. The risk of infection increases with the size of the wound. The risk of infection increases proportional to the length of time from injury to treatment of the wound.

Open fractures are graded as follows:

- Type I – A skin wound less than 1 cm that is clean.
- Type II – A skin wound more than 1 cm long, without extensive soft tissue damage, flaps or avulsions.
- Type III – A large wound with extensive skin and soft tissue contusion, muscle crush or loss. This grade is subdivided into:

  III(a) adequate soft tissue cover of the fractured bone despite extensive soft-tissue laceration or flaps;

  III(b) extensive soft tissue loss with periosteal stripping and bony exposure;

  III(c) an open fracture associated with an arterial injury requiring repair, irrespective of the degree of soft tissue injury.

Preoperative management

Preparation for surgery

Take microbiology swabs from the wound and cover the wound with a sterile dressing. Once covered, the wound should remain undisturbed until the patient reaches the operating theatre. Stop lots of people lifting off the dressing simply to view the wound. If you have access to a Polaroid camera, take a photograph of the wound and stick in the notes.

Treatment

Indications for surgery

All open wounds need debridement and irrigation within 6 hours of the accident. Bear in mind the time interval between the accident occuring and the patient arriving in casualty. The fracture has to be reduced and then immobilized.

Operation: irrigation and debridement of an open fracture

All contaminated and devitalized tissue is excised. If necessary the wound is extended to allow access to the damaged muscle. The wound is irrigated with copious amounts of saline. A pulsed lavage system may be used, but the pressure must be kept low to avoid forcing debris into the tissues rather than washing it out. In general the wound is not closed. Some surgeons may close a type I injury that is completely clean. The wound is then covered with swabs or a Vaseline impregnated gauge soaked in an aqueous antiseptic. The fracture is immobilized either in a plaster, by traction, or by an external fixator. In certain fractures, definitive internal fixation can safely be performed. This is only done by experienced surgeons. For example, an open fracture of the forearm should be treated with open reduction and internal fixation of the fractures combined with treatment of the soft tissues. An open fracture of the tibia can be fixed with an intra-medullary nail. If there is extensive soft tissue damage and the fracture needs to be fixed internally this can be done at the same operation. In many centres, the plastic surgeons work with the orthopaedic surgeons and will apply a flap to cover the wound once the fracture has been fixed.

When the wound has been left open, the patient is taken back to the operating theatre after 48 hours. Dead tissue is further debrided if necessary. If the wound is not infected, the wound should be closed. If there has been skin loss, you may need to involve the plastic surgeons to apply a split skin graft, a local flap or a free flap.

Codes

GA/LA	GA
Blood	Appropriate to fracture
Antibiotics	Yes
Time	Depends on wound
Drains	0
Plaster	Yes
Postoperative radiograph	Yes

Operative requirements

- A tourniquet should be applied, but only inflated if absolutely necessary.
- Pulsed lavage.

Postoperative care

Management

If the wound is left open, the patient will have to return to the theatre after 48 hours. Antibiotics should be continued until the wound is closed.

If the skin loss has been considerable, the wound may need to be covered with a split thickness skin graft or a local muscle flap.

If the wound is clean after 48 hours, internal fixation may be performed and the wound closed.

Complications

- Wound infection.
- Osteomyelitis.

Multiple trauma

It is not the role of the house officer to direct the initial management of the patient with multiple injuries. The principles and practice of the management of major trauma is taught on ATLS (Advanced Trauma Life Support) courses. Most hospitals follow the guidelines taught in ATLS. If you have not been on a course, study a course manual.

You will be involved in the initial care of patients with major trauma and you should remember the following:

Airway Ensure that the patient has an airway that is clear and not blocked by dentures, tongue or vomit.

Breathing If the patient is not breathing, you should not attempt to intubate the patient unless you have considerable experience. A properly applied face mask is usually better than spending time failing to intubate a patient.

Intravenous access Insert a cannula through which blood can be given. The smallest acceptable is a 16 gauge, but a 14 gauge is preferred. Insert two cannulae if possible. Take blood for cross match, full blood count and biochemistry when you insert the cannula.

Cross match If there is a significant injury, order blood to be cross matched and not just grouped and saved. If there is more than one injury, order enough blood. It is easy to underestimate what may be lost. If in doubt ask the senior person how much should be cross matched.

Radiographs The minimum that is required is a lateral view of the whole of the cervical spine, a chest radiograph, and an AP of the pelvis. These should be taken in the resuscitation room using the portable X-ray machine. Radiographs of an obviously fractured limb are not essential in the initial period of resuscitation.

Rheumatoid arthritis

The condition

This is a common disease that usually presents in middle age, and in women more than men. It is a systemic inflammatory disease that primarily affects synovial joints. It can affect most joints, both large and small. The pattern in which joints are affected varies considerably from patient to patient. Usually the pattern is similar for the patient's two sides.

Making the diagnosis

The patient
By the time a patient with rheumatoid arthritis presents to the orthopaedic department, the diagnosis is usually established.

The history
The rheumatoid patient often has an extensive medical and surgical history. However, there are several parts of the history you must elicit.

- How long has the patient had the disease and is it active or quiescent?
- How mobile is the patient?
- Which joints most limit the patient's activities?
- Which joint is the most painful?

Ask about each major joint in turn. First ask about pain and stiffness in the joint. Secondly, in your past surgical history, ask about operations to each joint. Try to include all procedures, in chronological order for each separate joint. You must ask about the shoulders, elbows, wrist, hands, hips, knees, ankles and feet.

Always ask the patient if they have a painful neck, since rheumatoid arthritis can lead to instability of the cervical spine. The disease can also affect the temporo-mandibular joints and make them stiff. This leads to a restricted jaw opening. Both of these points are important in regard to anaesthesia. Excessive movement of an unstable neck during intubation can injure the spinal cord. Intubation may be very difficult if the mouth cannot be opened wide due to stiff temporo-mandibular joints.

Take a drug history that includes the site and number of intra-articular steroid injections. Is the patient currently taking systemic steroids? If they are, the patient may require additional steroids in the perioperative period. Ask the patient if they have recently or are currently taking methotrexate. This cytotoxic is commonly used to treat rheumatoid arthritis. Most anaesthetists do not insist on stopping methotrexate prior to surgery, but some do. It is best to ask your consultant and the anaesthetist about the unit policy before the patient is admitted.

Take a careful social history. Does the patient live alone? If so, they may need additional social services once discharged from hospital. Do they have stairs to climb? If so, how many?

On examination

In a severe rheumatoid, a complete examination is a formidable task. It is best to be methodical and examine each joint in turn. Tabulate the findings in two columns, left and right. Place the 'right' column on the left, and the 'left' column on the right. This is easier to fill in, as this is the way that you look at the patient.

For each major joint, note any swelling, deformity, instability, range of movement and whether movement is painful throughout the range of movement or just at the end of the movement.

Radiographs

The signs of rheumatoid arthritis begin with diffuse porosis of the bones on *both* sides of the joint. The joint space becomes narrowed and finally the joint is destroyed. The joint may become subluxated or even dislocated.

Try to be selective in your request for radiographs.

Check the patient's packet to see when radiographs were last taken of the symptomatic joints. New views are only required if the interval is greater than 6 months, or if there has been a marked clinical deterioration since the last radiographs were taken.

Always ensure that there are views of the cervical spine.

Preoperative management

Investigations

Rheumatoid patients are often anaemic and have a raised erythrocyte sedimentation rate. Although often requested, the serological tests for rheumatoid arthritis are not very helpful in either diagnosis or treatment.

Treatment

The role of the physiotherapists, occupational therapists, social workers and nurses should not be underestimated in this debilitating, destructive disease. The initial treatment is always conservative. This includes resting a joint that is acutely inflamed either by bed rest or splints. In the non-inflamed state, joints are kept mobile with physiotherapy and home exercises.

Conservative treatment is usually supervised by the rheumatologists. The choice of anti-inflammatory medication ranges from aspirin, to non-steroidal anti-inflammatory drugs, to systemic cortico-steroids. Other drugs, such as gold and methotrexate are also used. Local cortico-steroids can be injected directly into an inflamed area and give good relief of pain. However, the injections cannot be given more than twice into any one site as there are risks of tendon rupture.

Indications for surgery

The main indication for surgery is pain. Joint stiffness alone is not an indication for surgery. Indeed a stiff but pain-free joint is a contra-indication to surgery and is the aim of an arthrodesis. Surgery may be indicated to correct deformity and improve function.

Surgical procedures include the following procedures:

Synovectomy, removal of the diseased synovium, is effective in some joints in reducing pain and slowing down joint destruction. Synovectomy around tendons may prevent tendon rupture.

Repair of ruptured tendons and soft tissue correction of deformities (especially in the hands), may considerably improve function.

Arthrodesis (fusion) of some joints may improve function in the adjacent joints by providing stability and reducing pain. Wrist fusion is a good example.

Joint replacement has a major role in the surgical treatment of rheumatoid arthritis. The relief of pain is predictable and the joints perform well. This is because the patients are less active than those with osteoarthritis. However, the risk of infection is higher in rheumatoid patients, especially if they are on systemic steroids.

Osteoarthritis

The condition

Osteoarthritis is the result of degeneration of the articular cartilage of a joint. If there is no known precipitating cause for the degeneration, then the osteoarthritis is considered to be primary. In most cases there is an identifiable cause for osteoarthritis. There may be an abnormality within the joint, such as previous intra-articular fracture or removal of the meniscus of the knee. Alternatively, there may be abnormal stresses through the joint – either excessive load as in obesity, or repetitive stress as in high-level sportsmen, or in an abnormal direction, such as following a fracture that has healed with an abnormal alignment.

Making the diagnosis

The patient

Most patients with osteoarthritis of a joint do not present until after middle age. However, if the degeneration follows a childhood problem (e.g. congenital dislocation of the hip), presentation may be as early as the second decade.

The history

You must take a careful history that extends as far back as the patient can recall. Patients often dismiss previous injuries as irrelevant if they occurred a long time in the past. Always enquire about the patient's previous occupation and hobbies. Ask about previous surgery to the limb.

As with any pain, ask about the site, nature, intensity, character, relieving factors, exacerbating factors and radiation. Assess the function of the joint by establishing how limited the patient is in his/her daily activities.

On examination

Look at the limb and the joint. Is there any deformity, muscle wasting or scarring? If the joint is enlarged, palpate the joint and decide if any swelling is bony due to osteophytes, or non-bony due to an effusion. Test the stability of the joint to see if the ligaments are intact. Establish the range of movement, both actively and passively. Is there a fixed deformity (that does not vary with the position of the joint)? Is there crepitus on moving the joint? Is the joint purely stiff, or is it pain that limits the joint's range of movement?

Radiographs

The first sign of osteoarthritis, loss of joint 'space' on the radiograph, reflects the fact that it is loss of articular cartilage that is the main pathology. This 'joint space' which is lost is, of course, the radiolucent articular cartilage. The later changes are osteophyte formation around the periphery of the joint, subchondral bone sclerosis (looks very white on the radiograph) and cyst formation.

Treatment

Conservative treatment should always be considered before surgery. Weight loss, change in occupation, use of a walking stick, mild analgesics and anti-inflammatory medication can all be effective. Physiotherapy may be useful in both relieving pain and increasing the range of movement.

The aim of surgery is primarily to relieve pain. Any gain in movement is purely an added bonus. A stiff but painless joint is a contra-indication to surgery. Surgical treatment includes arthrodesis, osteotomy and arthroplasty. Arthrodesis aims to produce a joint that is completely stiff, but pain free. Osteotomy realigns load transfer through a joint. The mechanism behind the success of osteotomies has not been completely explained but they can provide long-lasting pain relief. Neither arthrodesis nor osteotomy precludes later conversion to an arthroplasty.

Joint replacement is not possible for all joints and not ideal in the younger patients. There are major risks in the replacement of joints including infection, intraoperative and late bone fracture, failure of the components themselves and loosening of the components. Revision (reoperation) of joint replacement is always more difficult than the original operation and the results less predictable. However, when performed for the correct indications, joint replacement can transform a patient's life.

Infection in orthopaedics

One of the most serious complications following an orthopaedic operation is deep infection. The presence of a foreign body, even though sterile when inserted, can act as a nidus for infection. Once there is deep sepsis, the only way of removing the infection may be to remove the prosthesis.

The most common organism that infects prostheses is *Staphylococcus aureus*. However, *Staphylococcus epidermidis*, although regarded generally as non-pathogenic, can also cause deep infection.

In elective cases, when a prosthesis is to be inserted, the following measures should be taken:

1. On admission send a sample of midstream urine to microbiology for microscopy, culture and sensitivity. If the patient has a urinary tract infection, this should be treated prior to surgery.

2. The patient may have a bath or shower using an antiseptic soap, on the night before and on the day of surgery (not every unit does this).

3. The operation should be performed in a dedicated orthopaedic theatre. In many hospitals, the orthopaedic theatre has an ultra-clean air system of one sort or another. In some units the surgeon and assistants may operate wearing an exhaust suit that looks like a space suit. It is designed to carry away air from the surgeon's (dirty) body out of the operating field.

4. Because orthopaedic surgeons handle bone that has sharp and spiky edges, they usually operate wearing two pairs of gloves. This precaution means that if the outer glove is unknowingly perforated, the inner will

prevent possible contamination from the surgeon's skin. In addition, double gloving provides extra protection for the surgical team against infection from the patient. After prepping and draping the patient on the operating table, it is best to change the outer gloves, as they may have become contaminated. When the prosthesis itself is inserted, the surgeon should change his gloves for a new pair, in case he has unknowingly contaminated the first.

If at any time you feel that either you or the surgeon may have desterilized their gloves or gown, or an instrument or drape has become contaminated, you must inform the surgeon. No one will criticize you for trying to avert a disaster.

5. Whenever a prosthesis is inserted patients must receive antibiotic prophylaxis. This applies to artificial joints – both metal and plastic, screws, plates and intramedullary nails. Temporary K-wires do not need antibiotic cover. The commonest regime for prophylaxis is three intravenous doses of a second generation cephalosporin, such as cefuroxime. The first dose is given with induction of anaesthesia. If a tourniquet is used, the first dose of antibiotic should be given before the tourniquet is inflated. The second dose is given 8 hours after the first dose. The third dose, 16 hours after the first dose. If the patient is truly allergic to penicillin you can give a test dose of the cephalosporin to see if the patient is also allergic to that as well. If a cephalosporin cannot be used, give the patient three intravenous doses of erythromycin.

6. A patient who has a prosthesis must be given antibiotic cover if he is to undergo any further procedure that may result in a bacteraemia. If the patient requires a urinary catheter, you can prescribe oral trimethoprim while the catheter is *in situ*. Alternatively you can give an intramuscular dose of gentamicin 1 hour before the catheter is inserted and 1 hour before it is removed.

In trauma cases undergoing surgery, preoperative urine sample and antiseptic wash is often not possible, but the surgical techniques remain the same. For a closed fracture, the three dose cephalosporin regime is adequate. In open injuries, swabs should be taken from the wound and antibiotic therapy continued for a minimum of 48 hours (see Chapters 3 and 36).

Tetanus prophylaxis

For all patients with a wound, check that the patient is covered against tetanus:

1. A patient who has active immunity and received their last dose of tetanus toxoid within the last 5 years needs no further prophylaxis.

2. A patient whose last dose of toxoid was more than 5 years ago should be given a tetanus toxoid booster.

3. A patient who has never completed a tetanus toxoid course should commence one.

Compartment syndrome

The condition

Compartment syndrome occurs when pressure rises within a closed fascial space. This reduces the capillary perfusion below a level necessary for tissue viability. Intracompartmental pressure may become raised due to interstitial oedema, haemorrhage or muscle fibre swelling within the compartment. Compartment pressure may also become elevated by external constriction of the compartment (e.g. tight casts).

If a compartment syndrome is not effectively treated, the muscle within the compartment dies and fibroses. This results in a Volkmann's ischaemic contracture.

If a compartment syndrome is adequately treated, the limb will retain normal function.

Making the diagnosis

The patient

The patient may be acutely injured, having suffered a blow or crushing injury. Although a fracture may be present, it is the soft tissue injury that is important. Alternatively, the patient may have had an operation that involved considerable soft tissue trauma or was performed under a pneumatic tourniquet.

The history

The cardinal feature of a compartment syndrome is increasing pain, unrelieved by increased doses of analgesics. Later when the nerve that runs through the compartment becomes ischaemic, there will be paraesthesia and then numbness in the distribution of that nerve.

On examination

Stretching the muscles that are involved in the compartment syndrome increases the pain. When examining a patient who is at risk from a compartment syndrome, you must be gentle but thorough. In the upper limb with a forearm fracture, moving the fingers to a new position may be painful even without a compartment syndrome. What is significant, is if the discomfort/pain continues when the fingers are held extended without further movement. Similarly with the toes.

Since the major vessels have a greater pulse pressure than the microvascular circulation that is being compressed, one may find a palpable radial pulse at the wrist in the presence of a compartment syndrome. In short, the presence of a distal pulse does not exclude a compartment syndrome.

Examine the muscles of the leg or arm. In compartment syndrome, they may feel abnormally firm, and direct pressure is painful.

Examine sensation in the hand or the foot. If there is sensory disturbance, try to work out which nerve is affected.

Preoperative management

Investigations

The pressure in a compartment can be measured. However, lack of a means of measuring the compartment pressure should not detract from the clinical diagnosis and the need to operate.

Measurement can be done under local anaesthetic in casualty. The compartment pressure may be measured using a sphygmomanometer, a three-way tap and a saline column as used for measuring the central venous pressure. This is the Whiteside technique. Alternatively, there are hand-held devices that have a needle that is inserted into the compartment and which display the pressure in the compartment on a digital display.

In the forearm, you can measure the pressure in the deep and superficial compartments.

In the lower leg, the pressure in all four compartments – the superficial posterior, the deep posterior, the anterior and the lateral – should be measured. If the compartment pressure is greater than the diastolic blood pressure minus 30 mmHg, then a compartment syndrome is likely and urgent surgery is indicated.

Treatment

Indication for surgery
Clinical suspicion of a compartment syndrome.

Operation: decompressive fasciotomy for compartment syndrome

A true compartment syndrome is an emergency and time is of the essence.

In the forearm, a long curvilinear incision is made from the ante-cubital fossa down the radial side of the flexor muscles and across the wrist. The skin and all layers of the fascia are divided.

In the leg, the incisions depend upon which compartments are involved. The superficial and deep posterior compartments can be decompressed through a long posterior stocking-seam incision. The anterior and the lateral compartments can be reached through a single antero-lateral incision. Some surgeons prefer to decompress all four compartments through the single lateral incision.

In a true compartment syndrome, the muscles will bulge out through the fascia as it is cut and will look bruised and dusky. If there is a concomitant fracture, it is best fixed internally or stabilized with an external fixator. The open wound cannot be closed and is dressed. The patient will have to return to theatre for delayed closure of the wound once the muscle swelling has subsided. Complete closure of the skin is often impossible even after 10 days and the defect may need to be covered with a split skin graft.

Codes

GA/LA	GA
Blood	Group and save
Antibiotics	Yes
Time	30 minutes
Drains	0
Plaster	Sometimes
Stay	10 days
Follow-up	2 weeks
Off work	6 weeks minimum

Operative requirement
No tourniquet.

Postoperative care

Management
Gentle elevation of the limb.
Continue antibiotics while the wound is open.

Complications
- Wound infection.
- Incomplete fasciotomy or delayed fasciotomy resulting in a degree of late muscle contracture.

Deep venous thrombosis

The condition

Deep vein thrombosis is a common complication in orthopaedic patients. Most thromboses are subclinical and the diagnosis may only be made retrospectively with the appearance of the signs of venous incompetence. Following operations around the hip, at least a third of the patients develop a deep venous thrombosis, but only a minority become symptomatic. The thrombosis usually develops during surgery, but you must remember that many patients awaiting elective surgery are very inactive and may develop a thrombosis preoperatively.

Making the diagnosis

The patient

Deep vein thrombosis does not occur in children. The patient at risk is an adult who is immobilized on bed rest or who has a lower limb immobilized or has had an operation on the lower limb. Females who are taking the oral contraceptive pill are at a greater risk of developing a DVT following surgery. Presentation classically occurs at 7–10 days following surgery.

The history

The patient may complain of calf pain. However, most deep vein thromboses are pain free and clinically 'silent'. There may be a slight pyrexia and a mild tachycardia.

On examination

The clinical signs depend upon whether the thrombosis is confined to below the knee, or extends above the knee. A patient with a below-knee thrombosis will have calf tenderness and increased pain on dorsiflexion of the ankle. The calf may be measurably swollen. Acute thrombosis of the femoral or iliac veins leads to a grossly swollen leg and localized tenderness over the involved vein. It is often difficult to distinguish the mild oedema that occurs after any leg operation, from the swelling associated with a deep vein thrombosis. The two indicators of the latter are the pain and the time interval following surgery.

Management

Investigations
Patients at risk for developing a thrombosis can be screened using radioactive labelled fibrinogen, which is injected intravenously. A Geiger counter is used to make daily counts at predetermined levels in the limb. A localized increased uptake of fibrinogen may indicate a thrombosis and the patient should then have a venogram. This technique of screening with labelled fibrinogen is mainly used as a research technique.

If a patient is suspected of having a thrombosis, the veins can be examined using the portable Doppler ultrasound probe. The probe is placed over the popliteal vein and the femoral vein. Phasic flow in time with the respiration is normal and indicates that the vessel is patent. Squeezing the calf should produce a whoosh of flow if the veins are patent. If only high-pitched, non-phasic flow is heard, this may indicate early collateral venous flow. Alternatively, no flow may be heard. The Doppler is 90% accurate in the diagnosis of femoral thrombosis and above, but not so accurate below the popliteal fossa. Duplex ultrasound scanning by the radiologist is equally accurate in diagnosing the presence and location of a thrombosis.

The 'gold-standard' investigation for a suspected deep vein thrombosis is the venogram. Radio-opaque contrast is injected into a vein in the foot and the venous tree is imaged. If a femoral thrombosis is suspected, you must specifically request that the upper end of the clot is seen. This is because a clot extending into the iliac vein has a high risk of detaching and causing a pulmonary embolus. Some vascular surgeons recommend the insertion of an 'umbrella' in the inferior vena cava in this situation.

Prophylaxis

The policies for prophylaxis against deep vein thrombosis vary widely. The difficulty is in deciding who should receive prophylaxis and by what means.

Patients who are high risk include anyone having lower limb surgery or hip surgery, patients on prolonged bed rest, patients who have a plaster cast on the leg, patients who have a history of a previous deep vein thrombosis and females taking the oral contraceptive pill.

Mechanical prophylaxis used during surgery include putting a TED (thromboembolic deterrent) stocking on the unoperated leg or both legs, pneumatic boots, electrical calf stimulators and venous foot pumps. Postoperatively the patient may continue with TED stockings or the foot pumps.

Chemical prophylaxis measures include subcutaneous heparin 5000 units b.d., low dose warfarin maintaining a prothrombin ratio between 1.5 and 2, or low molecular heparin once or twice a day. If your patient is going to receive heparin or warfarin check his other medication. If he is on aspirin or non-steroidal anti inflammatory drugs, there is an increased risk of irritating ooze during surgery and also following surgery. Some consultants (myself included) instruct patients to stop taking non-steroidal anti-inflammatory drugs 10 days before a major operation in order to reduce postoperative wound problems.

In short it is best to find out the policy of your consultant for who receives deep vein thrombosis prophylaxis and by what means.

Treatment

Anticoagulation
Full anticoagulation of a postoperative patient has the risk of haematoma formation in relation to the wound. Full anticoagulation in the elderly has the risk of a cerebro-vascular accident due to an intra-cranial bleed. In the elderly, with a clot in the calf veins, the risk of a pulmonary embolism is small. Consequently, not all surgeons treat all deep vein thromboses. You should check with the surgeon before commencing full anticoagulation in the elderly, as once started it is difficult to stop.

Other relative contraindications to anticoagulation are a history of haematemesis, peptic ulceration, haematuria, hypertension and women in their first trimester or last 4 weeks of pregnancy.

Full anticoagulation with heparin of a symptomatic DVT gives considerable pain relief, and the swelling and redness usually settle within 48 hours.

If the diagnosis of a deep vein thrombosis is seriously being considered in a patient who would be treated should he have a thrombosis, but a venogram cannot be obtained until the next day (or after the weekend), treatment should be started immediately. If the venogram is normal the treatment can be discontinued.

Heparin

If the thrombosis is to be treated, start a continuous intravenous infusion of heparin in a dose of 100–150 i.u. per kg body weight every 6 hours. For most adults, a suitable regime would be 10,000 units intravenously as a loading dose followed by an infusion giving 30–40,000 units per day. Measure the KCCT after 4–6 hours, and then daily, aiming to keep it to two to three times the normal level.

Warfarin

Surgeons differ as to when they think that warfarin should be started. Some start it with the heparin, since it will take some days for the dose to stabilize. Some prefer to delay starting the warfarin for 5 days to allow the heparin to have full therapeutic effect. Warfarin takes 24–48 hours to have a measurable effect. Patients vary in their sensitivity to warfarin. The elderly and patients with a low body weight can be especially sensitive. Many drugs and conditions affect the activity of warfarin and you must be aware of possible interactions.

A therapeutic regime is to give a loading dose of 10 mg for two nights and then measure the prothrombin time ratio (patient's: standardized). The aim is to have a ratio between two and three. In many hospitals the haematologists will monitor the therapy, and even if they do not, they will be happy to advise on dosages. It is best to prescribe the warfarin to be given at 6 p.m. so that the results of the morning prothrombin ratio are available. If the patient has not suffered a DVT before and has undergone a procedure that can be identified as being high risk for developing a DVT, warfarin can probably be stopped after

3 months. However opinion is divided about the duration of anti-coagulation following a DVT or pulmonary embolus and you should ask your consultant about the unit policy.

Upper Limb

10 Dislocation of the acromio-clavicular joint

The condition

Injury to the acromio-clavicular joint is classified as:

Grade 1 – sprain. Only a few fibres of the acromio-clavicular ligament and the capsule are torn. The radiographs are normal and the diagnosis is purely clinical.

Grade 2 – subluxation. The joint capsule is ruptured but the coraco-clavicular ligaments are intact. The plain radiographs may show some subluxation of the distal end of the clavicle that is not obvious clinically

Grade 3 – complete dislocation. The coraco-clavicular ligaments (conoid and trapezoid) are completely ruptured. The distal end of the clavicle protrudes superiorly clinically and on the radiographs.

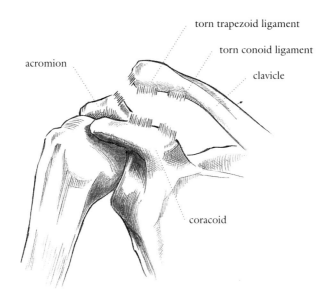

torn trapezoid ligament

torn conoid ligament

acromion

clavicle

coracoid

Making the diagnosis

The patient
The patient is usually an athletic male who has fallen directly onto the point of the shoulder. He usually points to the acromio-clavicular joint as the site of his pain.

On examination
The patient is tender over the acromio-clavicular joint. If it is a grade 3 injury, the outer end of the clavicle may be quite prominent.

Radiographs
Order an AP view of the shoulder. The radiograph of a patient with a pure ligamentous sprain is normal. A completely dislocated joint should be easily seen on an AP view of the shoulder. If there is any doubt as to the presence of a subluxation or dislocation, order 'weight-bearing' films of both the injured and the uninjured shoulder for comparison. These radiographs are taken with the patient holding a weight in each hand and may show a subluxation or dislocation more clearly.

Treatment

A broad arm sling and early mobilization is all that is necessary for grade 1 and grade 2 injuries. There is considerable debate about whether or not to operate on grade three dislocations acutely. Most surgeons feel that acute surgery is not indicated for the majority of patients. Most will become asymptomatic although the outer end of the clavicle may remain prominent. Acute open reduction and internal fixation is indicated for complete dislocation in the active young adult. such as a manual labourer or a high level sportsman.

Indications for surgery
Grade 3 injury in a young active patient (e.g. labourer or keen rugby player) may be an indication for surgery acutely.

If a patient has had a grade 3 injury many months previously and still has pain, we can perform surgery late. A ligament reconstruction is performed.

Operation: repair of acute dislocation of the acromio-clavicular joint

There are several methods of operative treatment of dislocation of the acromio-clavicular joint. The joint itself, as well as the coraco-clavicular ligament, have to be exposed. The incision can either be anterior over the delto-pectoral groove, or lateral. The joint is reduced under direct vision. It is held reduced either by a screw passing through the clavicle into the coracoid process (Bosworth screw), or by threaded pins that are passed through the acromion into the clavicle. The ligaments and the capsule also have to be repaired. The fixation, whether screw or pins, has to be removed after 6 weeks. This is because it would otherwise break once the patient starts moving his shoulder. The aim is simply to keep the dislocation reduced while the soft tissues heal.

Codes

GA/LA	GA
Blood	0
Antibiotics	Yes
Time	1 hour
Drains	0
Plaster	0
Postoperative radiograph	AP shoulder
Stay	24 hours
Follow-up	1 week
Off work	2–6 weeks depending on occupation

Operative requirements

Standard AO set, with a 4.5 mm lag screw or threaded pins.

Postoperative care

Management

The arm is rested in a broad arm sling for 1 week. Then gentle shoulder and elbow exercises are started, avoiding full elevation until the internal fixation is removed.

The patient is readmitted after 6 weeks for removal of the screw/pins as a day-case under GA.

Complications

- Injury to the brachial plexus.
- Redislocation following removal of the screw.
- Breakage of the pins or screws.

Operation: ligament reconstruction for chronic dislocation of the acromio-clavicular joint

There are several methods of operative treatment of chronic dislocation of the acromio-clavicular joint. The incision is anterior over the delto pectoral groove. The joint is reduced under direct vision. The coraco-acromial ligament is taken off the front of the acromion with a block of bone and transferred onto the clavicle. This recreates the coraco-clavicular ligament. A small screw holds the bone block in place. The clavicle is held reduced by a screw passing through the clavicle into the coracoid process (Bosworth screw). The Bosworth screw is removed after 6 weeks. This is because it would otherwise break once the patient starts moving his shoulder. The aim is simply to keep the dislocation reduced while the soft tissues heal.

Codes

GA/LA	GA
Blood	0
Antibiotics	Yes
Time	1 hour
Drains	0
Plaster	0
Postoperative radiograph	AP shoulder
Stay	24 hours
Follow-up	1 week
Off work	2–6 weeks depending on occupation

Operative requirements

Standard AO set, with a 4.5 mm lag screw and small fragment AO set.

Postoperative care

Management

The arm is rested in a broad arm sling for 1 week. Then gentle shoulder and elbow exercises are started, avoiding full elevation until the internal fixation is removed.

The patient is readmitted after 6 weeks for removal of the screw/pins as a day-case under GA.

Complications

- Injury to the brachial plexus.
- Redislocation following removal of the screw.
- Breakage of the pins or screws.

Investigation of the painful or unstable shoulder

The condition

There are many causes of shoulder pain. The patient may complain of an unstable shoulder and it can be difficult to work out whether there is true instability and in what direction the shoulder is unstable. If it is difficult to make a diagnosis on clinical features and radiological examination alone, an arthroscopy can be helpful.

Operation: arthroscopy of the shoulder

The arthroscope and a probe are inserted through 1 cm incisions, one posteriorly, one laterally just below the acromion and one anteriorly. The subacromial space can be seen as well as the shoulder joint itself.

Codes

GA/LA	GA
Blood	0
Antibiotics	0
Time	1 hour
Drains	0
Plaster	0
Postoperative radiograph	0
Stay	Day-case
Follow-up	10 days
Off work	10 days

Operative requirements

The patient is in the deck-chair position with a sand-bag under the shoulder or is on their side.

Postoperative care

Management

The patient goes home on the day of surgery. He should return to the outpatient department to have the dressings removed and the wound checked. The findings at arthroscopy are then discussed.

Complication

No diagnosis is made.

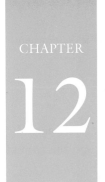

Dislocation of the shoulder

The condition

The most common dislocation of the head of the humerus is anterior, but it may dislocate posteriorly.

Making the diagnosis

The patient
The patient is typically a young adult but not necessarily so. Older patients can also suffer a dislocated shoulder.

The history
To dislocate a previously normal shoulder takes considerable force. The patient may recall falling or receiving a blow to the shoulder with the shoulder abducted beyond 90° and externally rotated. The patient has considerable pain around the shoulder and may suggest the diagnosis on arrival in casualty.

On examination
Look at both of the patient's shoulders. The normal contour of the dislocated shoulder is lost when compared with the uninjured one.

Test the function of the axillary nerve. Sensation is easy, i.e. sensation over the lateral part of the shoulder. Motor function is difficult to test with the shoulder dislocated. Ask the patient to try to gently abduct the shoulder while you palpate the deltoid muscle. If you feel any contraction within the deltoid, the motor supply is intact. Do not omit to also test the integrity of the median, ulnar and radial nerves.

Radiographs
An AP view of the shoulder will show the humeral head to be in an abnormal position. In an anterior dislocation, it lies inferior to the

coracoid. In a posterior dislocation, the head may look as if it is in the correct place, except that its orientation makes the head look like a light bulb.

Always ask for a second view. The easiest to interpret is an axillary view.

Common associated injuries

The axillary nerve may be injured when the shoulder dislocates or when it is reduced.

In patients over 50 years old, the rotator cuff may be torn.

Treatment

Indications for surgery

Acute dislocations of the shoulder need to be reduced. The sooner this is done the easier it is to do. The shoulder can be reduced in the Accident and Emergency department. If there is a humeral neck fracture as well as a dislocation, a closed reduction is often not possible and may result in injury to the axillary artery. Never try to reduce a dislocation associated with a humeral neck fracture under sedation in A&E.

Operation: reduction of dislocated shoulder

The shoulder can be reduced by a variety of techniques. Kocher's manoeuvre is most commonly used.

If the shoulder cannot be reduced under intravenous sedation, it is safer to ask an anaesthetist to give the patient a general anaesthetic, which provides complete relaxation. If you intend to reduce the shoulder under intravenous sedation, remember to maintain venous access and monitor the patient. Also remember that elderly patients can be very sensitive to sedatives and analgesics, and it is easy to inadvertently anaesthetize rather than sedate an elderly patient.

Codes

GA/LA	IV sedation or GA
Blood	0
Antibiotics	0
Time	10 minutes

Drains	0
Plaster	0
Postoperative radiograph	AP shoulder
Stay	Day case
Follow-up	3 weeks
Off work	3 weeks

Postoperative care

Management
Recheck the function of the axillary nerve after you have reduced the dislocation.

Always obtain post reduction radiographs.

In patients under 50 years old you should instruct the patient to rest the arm in a sling for 3 weeks before starting gentle active exercises. The patient must avoid external rotation combined with abduction for a total of 6 weeks. The aim is to allow the soft tissues to heal and reduce the likelihood of recurrent dislocations.

Since the risk of recurrent dislocation is very low in a patient over 50 years old, these patients are encouraged to regain full movement of the shoulder as quickly as possible. If an older patient complains of a lot of pain after 3 weeks following their shoulder dislocation, the rotator cuff may be torn. You should order an arthrogram of the shoulder to find out if the rotator cuff is intact.

Complications
- Axillary nerve injury.
- Humeral fracture during reduction.
- Rotator cuff tear.
- Recurrent dislocation.

CHAPTER

13

Recurrent dislocation of the shoulder

The condition

In a young adult, dislocation of the shoulder can tear the glenoid labrum and anterior capsule from its attachment on the front of the glenoid. This is called a Bankart lesion. This results in recurrent dislocation with little or no trauma.

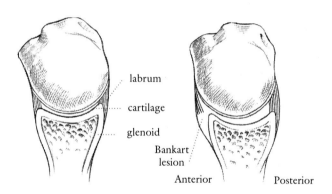

labrum

cartilage

glenoid

Bankart lesion

Anterior   Posterior

Making the diagnosis

The patient
The patient is typically a young adult male.

The history
The patient should have suffered an initial true dislocation of the shoulder, confirmed radiologically and requiring a doctor to reduce the shoulder. The radiographs will also show if the dislocation was anterior or posterior. The patient then suffers several more dislocations with much less trauma. Often the patient learns how to relocate his shoulder

himself. The patient will usually avoid placing their arm in the vulnerable position – shoulder abduction combined with external rotation.

The importance of this evidence is to confirm that there was indeed a dislocation as opposed to a feeling of the 'shoulder coming out of joint' that may be habitual subluxation. Patients with habitual subluxation do not need surgery.

On examination

Stand behind the seated patient. To examine the right shoulder, place your left hand on the patient's right shoulder with your middle finger on the coracoid process, your index finger on the front of the humeral head and your thumb behind the humeral head. Lift the patient's arm into abduction with external rotation. This will make the patient apprehensive and the humeral head will be felt to come forwards if there is true instability.

Document the integrity of the axillary nerve, i.e. intact sensation over the deltoid muscle and motor function of the deltoid, as the nerve can be damaged with dislocation.

Radiographs

Order AP and axillary views of both shoulders. A dent in the posterior part of the humeral head on the axillary view is a sign of recurrent anterior dislocation. The dent is caused by the front of the glenoid damaging the back of the humeral head when the shoulder is out of place.

Treatment

Indications for surgery

The indication for surgery is a history of multiple dislocations of the shoulder that interfere with the patient's daily activities.

If there is doubt about the diagnosis, open surgery may be preceded by arthroscopy of the shoulder. Damage to the back of the humeral head seen arthroscopically confirms that there have been several true anterior dislocations. At present it not possible to reliably stabilize a shoulder arthroscopically.

The patient must be made aware that following surgery there may be some loss of external rotation and that there will be a anterior scar.

Operation: stabilization of the shoulder for recurrent dislocation

The shoulder is exposed through an anterior bra-strap incision.

1. In the Bankart procedure, we correct the underlying lesion by reattaching the detached glenoid labrum to the glenoid.

2. In the Bristow procedure, the coracoid process is detached and reattached to the front of the glenoid to form a bony block to further anterior dislocation.

3. In the Putti-Platt operation, the subscapularis tendon and anterior capsule that run across the front of the shoulder are divided. They are tightened by being sutured back together in a double-breasted fashion.

Codes

GA/LA	GA
Blood	Group and save
Antibiotics	Optional
Time	1.5 hours
Drains	Occasionally
Plaster	0
Postoperative radiograph	0
Stay	1 days
Follow-up	10 days
Off work	6 weeks

Postoperative care

Management

Check the integrity of the musculo-cutaneous nerve by asking the patient to contract their biceps.

Elbow, wrist and hand exercises are started immediately.

The arm is held in a sling that prevents any external rotation for 6 weeks, and then the patient is allowed to self-mobilize.

Complications

- Neuro-vascular injury, especially to the musculo-cutaneous nerve.
- Recurrent dislocation (approximately 5%).

14

Subacromial bursitis

The condition

The rotator cuff is the group of tendons over the top of the humeral head that moves the arm. Between the acromion and coraco-acromial ligament above, and the rotator cuff below, is the subacromial bursa.

The subacromial bursa can become inflamed. This is due to the rotator cuff impinging on the anterior part of the acromion and the coraco-acromial ligament. This results in pain on performing certain movements, such as raising the arm above shoulder height.

Subacromial bursitis is also known as impingement syndrome or painful arc syndrome.

Making the diagnosis

The patient
Subacromial bursitis typically occurs in middle-aged and late middle-aged patients.

The history
There is usually no history of trauma or a trigger event. Sometimes the patient may recall falling onto the shoulder or outstretched hand. The patient may have overused the shoulder when painting a ceiling or playing an excessive amount of tennis. They complain of pain on trying to do anything with the arm elevated, such as combing their hair or getting something off a high shelf.

On examination
Examine both shoulders and compare the movements of the two sides. Document the full range of active flexion, abduction, external rotation and internal rotation.

The patient with subacromial bursitis typically has a painful arc. This is when abduction up to a point is pain free, and then the patient has pain on further abduction. Occasionally they then have no pain in the last part of abduction. They may have a painful arc during flexion, but the arc may be higher in the movement than the painful arc during abduction.

Assess the integrity of the rotator cuff by testing the power of external rotation, internal rotation and abduction.

On initial presentation in the outpatient clinic, the diagnosis can be confirmed by injecting some local anaesthetic into the subacromial space. It is important to explain to the patient that the injection is a test to see if the local anaesthetic eliminates their painful arc. 2 ml of 1% lignocaine is adequate. If the patient says that the majority of their pain on abduction is eliminated by the injection, then they probably do have subacromial bursitis.

Radiographs
Plain radiographs must be obtained, but are not very helpful. You can ask for special views to show the anterior end of the acromion.

An arthrogram will prove whether or not the rotator cuff is torn.

An MR scan can show fluid in the subacromial space that suggests that there is inflammation. The scan can also demonstrate a rotator cuff tear or degenerative change in the acromio-clavicular joint.

Fluid in the subacromial space can also be demonstrated with an ultrasound. However the reliability of the ultrasound depends on the experience of the ultrasonographer.

Treatment

The majority of patients are treated conservatively. Treatment includes non-steroidal anti-inflammatory medication, injection of local steroid into the subacromial space and physiotherapy. The local steroid injection may only relieve the pain for a few months or it may give permanent relief. The injection can be repeated on two occasions.

Indications for surgery
A positive diagnosis of subacromial bursitis and failure of conservative treatment.

Operation: open subacromial decompression

The incision is 10 cm long in the line of a bra strap at the front of the shoulder. The deltoid muscle is split. The coraco-acromial ligament is divided and the anterior overhanging part of the acromion is removed. This gives more room for the rotator cuff and prevents impingement.

Codes

GA/LA	GA
Blood	Group and save
Antibiotics	0
Time	1 hour
Drains	0
Sling	Yes
Postoperative radiograph	0
Stay	2 nights post operation
Follow-up	10 days
Off work	Light work 3 weeks
	Manual work 3 months

Operative requirements
The patient is in the deck-chair position with a sand-bag under the shoulder. A saw is used to remove the bone.

Postoperative care

Management
The patient must have intensive physiotherapy immediately following surgery. They should be able to fully abduct the operated arm with help from their other arm by the time they go home. You must give adequate analgesics and anti-inflammatories for them to be able to perform their exercises. The patient must have outpatient physiotherapy immediately following discharge.

Complications
Neuro-vascular damage; the axillary nerve is most at risk but injury is very rare. Persistent stiffness requiring a manipulation under anaesthetic. Wound infection.

Operation: arthroscopic subacromial decompression

The arthroscope and the powered shaver are inserted through 1 cm incisions, one posteriorly and one laterally just below the acromion. The coraco-acromial ligament is divided and the anterior overhanging part of the acromion shaved off. This gives more room for the rotator cuff and prevents impingement.

Codes

GA/LA	GA
Blood	0
Antibiotics	0
Time	1 hour
Drains	0
Sling	Yes
Postoperative radiograph	0
Stay	1 night post operation
Follow-up	10 days
Off work	Light work 3 weeks
	Manual work 3 months

Operative requirements

The patient is either in the deck-chair position with a sand-bag under the shoulder or is on their side. Traction is used to maintain distraction on the arm to pull the humeral head and rotator cuff away from the acromion. A special pump is required to pump irrigation fluid (normal saline) in at a constant pressure so the surgeon can see what he is doing. A powered shaver is used to remove bone and ligament.

Postoperative care

Management

The patient's shoulder is often quite swollen immediately following surgery due to fluid being pumped into the soft tissue. The swelling usually goes within 2 days.

The patient must have intensive physiotherapy immediately following surgery. They should be able to fully abduct the operated arm with help from their other arm by the time they go home. You must give adequate analgesics and anti-inflammatories for them to be able to perform their exercises. The patient must have outpatient physiotherapy immediately following discharge.

Complications
- Persistent stiffness requiring a manipulation under anaesthetic.
- Wound infection.
- Inadequate decompression.

15

Tear of the rotator cuff of the shoulder

The condition

The rotator cuff is made up of the tendons of supraspinatus, infraspinatus and teres minor. The tendons run over the top of the humeral head and beneath the acromion and coraco-acromial ligament. Tears occur in a cuff that is degenerate. There may be a history of an acute event such as a fall or dislocation of the shoulder. Alternatively, there may not be an acute precipitating event.

Making the diagnosis

The patient
The patient is usually middle-aged.

The history
The patient often injures the shoulder while protecting him/herself in a fall. If the patient feels that they have only suffered a sprain, they may not seek a medical opinion until months later when the symptoms have failed to settle. The typical picture is a patient who cannot actively abduct beyond 20–30°. They complain of not being able to reach up for things on a shelf or to brush their hair. Some patients are less typical and present with pain without dramatic weakness.

On examination
Examine both shoulders and compare the movements of the two sides. Document the full range of active and passive flexion, abduction, external rotation and internal rotation. Assess the integrity of the rotator cuff by testing the power of external rotation, internal rotation and abduction of both shoulders.

If the patient has a lot of pain it may be difficult to assess the power of the rotator cuff. In the outpatient department the diagnosis can be confirmed by injecting some local anaesthetic into the subacromial space. It is important to explain to the patient that the injection is a test to see if the local anaesthetic eliminates their pain. 2 ml of 1% lignocaine is adequate. If the majority of their pain is eliminated by the injection but they still have reduced power of abduction or external rotation, then they probably do have a torn rotator cuff.

A patient with a large tear of the rotator cuff may demonstrate *active* abduction that is markedly reduced. However, you should be able to passively abduct the arm past 90°. At this point the patient may be able to keep the arm raised by using their deltoid.

Radiographs

Order an AP view of the shoulder. Avulsion of the greater tuberosity of the humeral head is pathognomonic of a torn rotator cuff. This is seen with the minority of torn cuffs.

In patients who are seen after the acute event, a plain AP radiograph may show a diminished space between the humeral head and the acromion. This suggests that the cuff is torn and no longer separates the humeral head from the acromion. If in doubt, obtain a view of the normal side for comparison.

The definitive investigation is the double contrast arthrogram. If there is a tear, the contrast is seen to pass out of the shoulder joint into the subacromial bursa.

The rotator cuff is clearly seen on an MR scan. The accuracy in detection of full thickness tears depends on the both the scanner and the radiologist.

Treatment

Indications for surgery

A complete tear of the rotator cuff demonstrated on the arthrogram or MR scan, in a patient who has pain and/or weakness.

Operation: repair of the torn rotator cuff of the shoulder

Some surgeons approach the shoulder through a vertical but lateral incision that splits the acromion. Others prefer a bra-strap incision that runs over the delto-pectoral groove. The cuff is mobilized and repaired. This can be difficult in a cuff that is very degenerate.

Codes

GA/LA	GA
Blood	Group and save
Antibiotics	Yes
Time	1 hour
Drains	0
Plaster	0
Postoperative radiograph	0
Stay	3–5 days
Follow-up	3 weeks
Off work	8 weeks

Operative requirements
The patient should be in the deck-chair position with a sand-bag under the shoulder that is being operated upon.

Postoperative care

Management
The arm should be rested in a sling that includes a circumferential body strap to prevent external rotation of the arm. When the pain has subsided, gentle pendulum exercises are begun. The physiotherapist should help the patient perform passive movements. The patient is taught to use their unoperated arm to lift their operated arm into full elevation. Obviously if the patient tries to lift the operated arm *actively*, they may pull the tendon repair apart.

After 6 weeks active assisted exercises are begun.

Complications
- Neuro-vascular damage.
- Wound infection.
- Re-rupture.
- Stiffness.

Arthritis of the shoulder

The condition

Severe arthritis of the shoulder is common in patients with rheumatoid arthritis. Primary osteoarthritis of the shoulder is uncommon, but secondary osteoarthritis can follow trauma to the shoulder.

Making the diagnosis

The patient
The patient usually has polyarticular rheumatoid arthritis involving other upper limb joints.

The history
The most significant symptom is pain. This is usually accompanied by stiffness. Daily activities such as brushing the hair or getting the hand to the mouth may be impossible. You should also ask whether the patient can perform 'personal hygiene' after going to the toilet.

Ask the patient about their other joints and try and establish which of their upper limb joints is most troublesome. Also try and work out whether it is pain or stiffness which is causing the functional problem.

On examination
Examine the active range of movement of the shoulder. Fix the scapula with one hand whilst assisting with the range of movements to distinguish between scapulo-thoracic and gleno-humeral movement.

Examine the upper limbs in total, as other more severely affected joints may require surgery first.

Radiographs
AP and axillary views of the shoulder.

Preoperative management

Preparation for surgery
If the patient has rheumatoid arthritis, examine the range of neck and temporo-mandibular movements.

Ensure that there are a recent set of cervical spine radiographs to exclude cervical instability.

Treatment

Indications for surgery
Severe pain in the shoulder that is unrelieved by conservative measures, i.e. physiotherapy and intra-articular steroid injections.

Operation: total shoulder replacement

We make an anterior bra-strap incision and divide the subscapularis tendon and the anterior capsule. The articular surface of the humeral head is removed, and a metal humeral prosthesis, similar to the femoral component of a total hip replacement, is inserted down the shaft of the humerus. The glenoid may or may not be replaced. The glenoid component is either totally plastic or metal backed, depending on the design of the prosthesis. The components can be inserted with or without cement.

Codes

GA/LA	GA
Blood	Group and save
Antibiotics	Yes
Time	1.5 hours
Drains	Yes
Plaster	0
Postoperative radiograph	AP and lateral shoulder
Stay	10 days
Follow-up	6 weeks
Off work	3 months

Operative requirements
Arrange the patient in the astronaut/deck-chair position, with a sand-bag under the shoulder to be operated upon.

Postoperative care

Management
Check the integrity of the median, radial and ulnar nerves. The upper limb is rested in a sling for 5 days. Gentle mobilization is then commenced. The patient can be discharged home when they can touch their nose and when they can hold a cup of tea.

Complications
- Nerve injury.
- Infection.
- Dislocation.
- Loosening.

Fracture of the head and neck of the humerus

Making the diagnosis

The patient
The patient is typically middle-aged or elderly.

The history
The fracture usually results from a low velocity injury such as a simple fall.

On examination
A severe injury to the shoulder is usually obvious.

Examine the contour of the shoulder to see if the humeral head is dislocated as well as fractured.

Radiographs
Good quality radiographs are essential. The AP view should ideally be taken with the arm dependent to reduce the displacement of the fracture fragments. This makes evaluation of the fracture pattern easier. Ask the radiographer to take the radiograph with the patient sitting or standing (but not lying), and wearing their collar and cuff.

Ask for a shoot through or axial view to see if the humeral head is dislocated.

Preoperative management

Preparation for surgery
Rest the arm in a collar and cuff.

Treatment

The majority of patients with fracture of the humeral neck are managed as outpatients. The arm is rested in a collar and cuff. The elbow must not be supported either in a triangular sling nor supported by a well intentioned pillow. The idea of the collar and cuff is to allow gravity to help maintain the fracture in a satisfactory position. After three weeks the fracture is sticky enough for you to instruct the patient to begin moving their shoulder. If necessary refer the patient for physiotherapy.

Indication for surgery
A fracture of the upper humerus with several fragments that are displaced.

Operation: shoulder replacement (hemiarthroplasty)

The incision is in the line of a bra-strap incision anteriorly. The interval between deltoid and pectoralis is opened and the subscapularis tendon is divided.

The articular surface of the humeral head is removed. The greater tuberosity is preserved to allow attachment of the rotator cuff to the prosthesis and humeral shaft. A metal humeral prosthesis, similar to the femoral component of a total hip replacement, is inserted down the shaft of the humerus. The glenoid is not replaced. The prosthesis is inserted with or without cement.

Codes
GA/LA	GA
Blood	Group and save
Antibiotics	Yes
Time	1.5 hours
Drains	Yes
Plaster	0
Postoperative radiograph	AP shoulder
Stay	10 days
Follow-up	6 weeks
Off work	3 months

Operative requirements
Arrange the patient in the astronaut/deck-chair position, with a sand-bag under the shoulder to be operated upon.

Postoperative care

Management
Check the integrity of the median, radial and ulnar nerves.

Gentle passive mobilization starts after 5 days with the help of the physiotherapist. Exact instructions should be given by the surgeon.

The patient can be discharged home when they can touch their nose and when they can hold a cup of tea.

Complications
- Nerve injury.
- Infection.
- Dislocation.
- Loosening.

18

Fracture of the shaft of the humerus

Making the diagnosis

The patient

In the young adult, considerable force is required to break the humerus. In the older patient a fracture can occur with minimal trauma. Remember that the humerus is a common site for secondary deposits and a fracture may be a pathological fracture.

The history

The patient may have suffered a direct blow on the upper arm, may have fallen onto the arm or have been in a road traffic accident.

On examination

The diagnosis of the fracture itself is usually obvious. Examine the contour of the shoulder to exclude an associated dislocation.

Examine the function of the radial nerve; i.e. sensation over the dorsum of the hand, and active wrist dorsiflexion and metacarpophalangeal joint extension.

Radiographs

Ensure that the whole humerus has been X-rayed. Both the shoulder and the elbow must be included.

Preoperative management

Common associated injuries

Radial nerve neurapraxia or division.

Preparation for surgery

Depending on the instability of the fracture and the time until surgery, immobilize the arm in either a U-slab or just a collar and cuff.

Treatment

The majority of isolated humeral shaft fractures can be managed as an outpatient in a collar and cuff. Once the swelling has subsided, you should give your patient a humeral brace to wear.

Indications for surgery
Patient with multiple injuries.

Unacceptable position of fracture after a trial of conservative therapy in a collar and cuff or plaster immobilization.

Delayed/non-union.

If the radial nerve ceases to function either immediately following the fracture, or after manipulation of the fracture, the nerve should be explored and repaired if necessary. The fracture has to be stabilized in order to allow the nerve to be repaired.

Operation: internal fixation of fractured shaft of humerus

The precise method of fixation depends on the fracture and the surgeon. The choice is either open plating of the fracture or closed reduction and insertion of an intramedullary nail. The nail can either be inserted from above, through the non-articular part of the humeral head, or from below, through the olecranon fossa.

Codes
GA/LA	GA
Blood	Group and save
Antibiotics	Yes
Time	1.5 hours
Drains	Yes
Plaster	0
Postoperative radiograph	AP and lateral humerus
Stay	3–4 days
Follow-up	10 days
Off work	8 weeks

Operative requirements

If a closed procedure (insertion of an intramedullary nail) is to be performed, then the image intensifier and a radiographer are required.

Postoperative care

Management

Check the integrity of the radial nerve in recovery.

Encourage the patient to mobilize the whole limb if the fixation is stable and a nerve repair has not been performed. Otherwise, immobilize the upper limb with an above elbow cast for 3–6 weeks.

Complications

- Permanent or temporary injury to the radial nerve.
- Infection.
- Inadequate fixation.
- Non-union.

Supracondylar fracture of the humerus

The condition

A fracture of the distal humerus that may, or may not, extend into the elbow joint.

Making the diagnosis

The patient

This fracture is common in children who fall onto the outstretched arm. The fracture is often minimally displaced and is not usually comminuted.

By contrast, this fracture is uncommon in adults, when it often occurs as a result of a high energy injury such as a fall from a height or a motorcycle accident.

On examination

The elbow may be grossly swollen. Examine and document the presence of the radial pulse and the intact function of the radial, median and ulnar nerves.

Radiographs

Order AP and lateral views of the whole humerus. It is essential in children and often helpful in adults to ask for radiographs of the uninjured elbow for comparison.

Preoperative management

Common associated injuries

Entrapment or division of the brachial artery.

Preparation for surgery

Place the arm in an above-elbow back-slab with the arm in whatever position is most comfortable, until the patient goes to theatre. Make sure that the radial pulse is still present after the back-slab has been applied.

Treatment

Treatment of children's fractures

An operation is not indicated for a child with an undisplaced crack, or a fracture that is angulated less than 20° on the lateral view. Simply immobilize the child's arm in an above-elbow back-slab with a collar and cuff, or even just a collar and cuff. The choice depends on how much pain the child is in. The cast and/or collar and cuff is kept on for 3 weeks. The arm is then left free of any immobilization. Children do not generally require physiotherapy.

A fracture that is only angulated on the lateral view of the elbow can usually be manipulated into a satisfactory position.

If a displaced fracture can be reduced, but once reduced seems unstable, the position may be held with K-wires. These are left protruding through the skin for ease of removal.

If the fracture cannot be reduced closed, an open reduction may be necessary, and this possibility must be included on the consent.

If the fracture cannot be reduced and the arm is very swollen, the arm should be put on traction using either skin traction or a traction screw inserted into the coronoid process of the ulna.

Treatment of adult fractures

Unless truly undisplaced, most supracondylar fractures require open reduction and internal fixation.

Indications for surgery

Displaced fracture.
Comminuted fracture that can be reconstructed.

Operation: manipulation under anaesthesia of supracondylar fracture of the humerus in a child

The arm is manipulated and the position is checked with the image intensifier. The arm should be immobilized in a collar and cuff with the elbow flexed. Since excessive flexion can occlude the brachial artery, the degree of elbow flexion is a compromise between stability and vascularity. Many surgeons feel that if an operation is needed, the fracture should be stabilized with percutaneous K-wires to prevent loss of position and the need for a further operation.

Codes

GA/LA	GA
Blood	0
Antibiotics	0
Time	30 minutes
Drains	0
Plaster	Above elbow
Postoperative radiograph	AP and lateral elbow
Stay	2 nights
Follow-up	1 week, X-ray on arrival
Off school	2 weeks

Operative requirements
Image intensifier and radiographer.

Postoperative care

Management
The major risk following manipulation of this fracture is the development of a compartment syndrome. Carefully check the movement of the fingers. Loss of full extension of the fingers due to pain is the first sign of a compartment syndrome. If the child has increasing pain, do not just give stronger analgesics, but carefully assess the child and if at all concerned, call a more senior person.

Complications
- Compartment syndrome.
- Loss of position.
- Abnormal growth leading to a gun-stock deformity.

Operation: open reduction and K-wiring of supracondylar fracture of the humerus in a child

The fracture is reduced through a lateral incision plus/minus a medial incision. Once reduced, two K-wires are inserted. The reduction and the position of the wires is checked with the image intensifier.

Codes

GA/LA	GA
Blood	0
Antibiotics	Yes
Time	1 hour
Drains	0
Plaster	Above-elbow back-slab
Postoperative radiograph	AP and lateral elbow
Stay	3 days
Follow-up	1 week
Off school	2 weeks

Operative requirements

- K-wires and Jacob's chuck.
- Radiographer and image intensifier.

Postoperative care

Management

The major risk following open reduction of this fracture is the development of a compartment syndrome. Carefully check the sensation and movement of the fingers. If the child has increasing pain, do not just give stronger analgesics, but carefully assess the child and if at all concerned, call a more senior person.

Complications

- Compartment syndrome.
- Loss of position.
- Abnormal growth leading to a gun-stock deformity.

Operation: insertion of olecranon skeletal traction screw for supracondylar fracture of the humerus in a child

A small incision is made over the ulna opposite the coronoid process. A screw is inserted perpendicular to the long axis of the ulna, to which traction is attached.

Codes

GA/LA	GA
Blood	0
Antibiotics	0
Time	30 minutes
Drains	0
Stay	2 weeks
Postoperative radiograph	AP and lateral elbow in traction
Follow-up	1 week, X-ray on arrival

Operative requirements

- Small fragment AO malleolar screw.
- Set up the traction on the bed prior to the procedure so that the patient can be placed on traction while anaesthetized.

Postoperative care

Management

Beware compartment syndrome – if the patient has increasing pain, and the fingers cannot be passively extended, call a senior person. Do not just give stronger analgesics.

Arrange longitudinal traction on the ulna with 1.5–2.5 kg (3–5 lb) from the screw, and skin traction on forearm to maintain the elbow at approximately 45° with 0.5–1 kg (1–2 lb).

Traction is maintained for 2 weeks and then the patient is discharged home in an above-elbow plaster in which they remain for one further week.

Complications

- Compartment syndrome.
- Loss of position.

■ Abnormal growth; a varus deformity is the commonest and cosmetically most unacceptable deformity.

Operation: open reduction and internal fixation of supracondylar fracture of the humerus in an adult

A midline posterior incision is used. If the fracture involves the articular surface of the distal humerus, it is vital that the joint is reconstructed as perfectly as is possible. To do this, we may osteotomise (divide) the olecranon to permit the triceps insertion to be elevated. This manoeuvre provides a clear view of the distal humerus. The fracture fragments are reduced and then held with plates and screws. The olecranon is held with a single large screw.

Codes

GA/LA	GA
Blood	0
Antibiotics	Yes
Time	1–1.5 hours
Drains	Yes
Plaster	Above elbow
Postoperative radiograph	AP and lateral elbow
Stay	3 days
Follow-up	2 weeks
Off work	6 weeks

Operative requirements

K-wire set, small AO and standard AO sets, small reconstruction plates and small cannulated screws.

Tourniquet high on the upper arm.

Some surgeons prefer to check the reduction in theatre with an on-table radiograph or with the image intensifier. If so, warn the radiographer.

Postoperative care

Management

If the fixation is solid, gentle active mobilization can begin immediately. Otherwise, the arm is kept in the back-slab for 3 weeks.

Complications
- Failure to achieve anatomical reduction.
- Injury to the ulnar or radial nerve. This is commonly a neurapraxia that can take several months to recover. Rarely a nerve may be divided.
- Failure of fixation.
- Stiffness.
- Wound infection.
- Late osteoarthritis.

CHAPTER 20

Tennis elbow

The condition

Tennis elbow is the colloquial name for lateral epicondylitis. The cause of the inflammation is often not clear. A repetitive activity that stresses the extensor muscles of the forearm can trigger off lateral epicondylitis.

Making the diagnosis

The history

Tennis elbow is characterized by pain that is maximal over the lateral epicondyle of the elbow. There will have been a gradual onset of pain that occurs with certain movements and may radiate down the whole forearm.

Ask the patient if they have abnormal sensation down the radial side of the forearm. If they do, they may have entrapment of the radial nerve and not a simple tennis elbow.

On examination

The area of tenderness is over the lateral epicondyle.

Stretching the patient's extensor muscles by extending the elbow, and palmar flexing the wrist is painful. This pain is increased by asking the patient to maintain this position against resistance.

Radiographs

AP and lateral views of the elbow are necessary to exclude an alternate cause for the pain. The radiographs are usually normal.

Treatment

The majority of patients are made comfortable with conservative treatment and do not require surgery. Treatment options include physiotherapy, local injection of lignocaine and steroid, a course of a non-steroidal anti-inflammatory drug and use of a tennis elbow band.

A steroid injection should only be performed two or three times. The patient should be warned that there is a risk that they may suffer local skin changes as a result of an injection. The skin can lose some of its colour and also become thin due to loss of underlying fat.

If the patient is a sports enthusiast and has become comfortable with conservative treatment, he should be told to warm up properly before playing sport. The patient must pay particular attention to stretching the forearm extensor muscles.

Indications for surgery
Persistent or recurrent pain that has failed to respond to conservative treatment.

Operation: release of the extensor origin for tennis elbow

A curved incision is made on the lateral side of the elbow. The origin of the extensor muscles is elevated from the bone and allowed to heal in a slightly more distal position.

Codes
GA/LA	GA
Blood	0
Antibiotics	0
Time	30 minutes
Drains	0
Plaster	Above elbow removable cast or brace
Postoperative radiograph	0
Stay	Day case
Follow-up	2 weeks
Off work	2 weeks

Operative requirement
Above-elbow tourniquet.

Postoperative care

Management

Check the integrity of the posterior interosseous nerve – can the patient actively dorsiflex their wrist?

Encourage finger mobilization.

Some surgeons keep the patient's elbow immobile for 2 weeks in the plaster cast. Others begin supervised exercises after 2 days following surgery. In between exercises, the elbow is rested in the plaster or brace.

Complications

The posterior interosseous nerve is at risk and may be bruised or even divided, leading to a wrist drop.

21

Fracture of the olecranon

The condition

A fracture of the olecranon usually extends into the elbow joint, and is in essence an avulsion fracture of the triceps insertion. The proximal fragment usually displaces proximally, due to the pull of the triceps. The fracture is an intra-articular fracture.

Making the diagnosis

The history

This fracture commonly occurs in patients in or beyond their middle age, but not always. The history is of a fall onto the point of the elbow.

On examination

There is considerable bruising and swelling around the elbow. Test the ability of the patient to actively extend the elbow. Active extension is absent in displaced fractures.

It is important to examine and document the integrity of ulnar nerve sensation (ulnar one and a half fingers) and motor function (finger abduction).

Radiographs

AP and lateral of the elbow.

Preoperative management

Preparation for surgery

The arm must be rested, prior to surgery, in a well-padded back-slab with the elbow at 90°.

Treatment

Indications for surgery
A displaced fracture.

Operation: tension band wiring of fractured olecranon

A midline posterior incision is used. The fragments are reduced and then held with two K-wires inserted longitudinally and a crossed wire loop. The aim of the wire loop is to increase the compression on the fracture when the elbow is flexed – hence 'tension band' wiring. Since this is an intra-articular fracture, the surgeon should try to achieve an anatomical reduction of the joint surface.

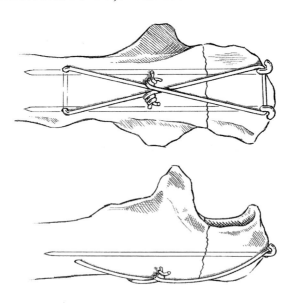

Codes

GA/LA	GA
Blood	0
Antibiotics	Yes
Time	1 hour
Drains	Yes
Plaster	Above elbow
Postoperative radiograph	AP and lateral elbow

Stay	3 days
Follow-up	2 weeks
Off work	4 weeks

Operative requirements

- K-wire set.
- Tourniquet high on upper arm.
- Some surgeons prefer to check the reduction in theatre with an on-table radiograph or with the image intensifier. If so, warn the radiographer.

Postoperative care

Management

If the fracture fixation is solid, gentle active mobilization can begin immediately. Otherwise, the arm is kept in the back-slab for 3 weeks.

Complications

- Failure to achieve anatomical reduction.
- Division of the ulnar nerve.
- Failure of fixation.
- Late arthritis (the risk of degenerative change increases if the reduction is not anatomical).

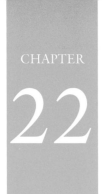

Fracture of the radial head

Making the diagnosis

The history

The patient has usually fallen onto the outstretched hand and will complain of pain around the elbow. Sometimes the pain is surprisingly mild. Sometimes it is quite severe.

On examination

Feel for tenderness over the radial head.

Examine the range of pronation and supination, which may be restricted by pain. If the patient has severe pain and a restricted range of pronation and supination, you should perform an examination under anaesthetic. This is easily done in the casualty or fracture clinic.

Ask the patient to lie on an examination couch on their side, with the injured elbow uppermost. Palpate and mark out the prominences of the radial head, the lateral epicondyle and the tip of the olecranon. Prepare a sterile trolley including a syringe containing 5 ml of 1% ligno-caine and an empty 10 ml syringe. Using an aseptic no-touch technique, infiltrate 1 ml of lignocaine into the skin into the middle of the triangle formed by the bony landmarks. Insert a green needle on the empty syringe until you aspirate haematoma. Withdraw as much of the haematoma as possible and then take the syringe off the needle. Leave the needle in the joint so as not to loose your position. Inject the rest of the lignocaine into the joint. After a few minutes you should be able to move the elbow without hurting the patient. If there is a full range of supination and pronation, surgery cannot improve things, whatever the fracture looks like on the radiograph.

If the patient is in severe pain, aspiration of the haemarthrosis will greatly relieve the patient's agony.

Radiographs

If a fracture is suspected, ask for AP and lateral views of the elbow as well as oblique 'radial head views'.

Preoperative management

Preparation for surgery

Rest the elbow in a well-padded back-slab prior to surgery.

Treatment

Undisplaced fractures can be rested in an above-elbow back-slab for 1 or 2 weeks, prior to beginning mobilization.

Indications for surgery

A displaced fracture with a block to rotation of the forearm when examined under local anaesthesia.

Operation: open reduction and internal fixation of a fractured radial head

The fracture is exposed through a lateral incision centred over the radial head. If possible, the fragments are reduced and then held using mini-fragment screws. The aim is to reconstruct the joint surface. If the fracture is so comminuted that reconstruction is not possible, the radial head may have to be excised. The patient should be aware of this possibility. Some surgeons like to put in an artificial replacement if the radial head is removed. This acts as a spacer and maintains the correct relationship between the radius and ulna.

Codes

GA/LA	GA
Blood	0
Antibiotics	Yes
Time	1 hour
Drains	0
Plaster	Above elbow
Postoperative radiograph	AP and lateral elbow
Stay	2 days

Follow-up   10 days

Off work   3 weeks minimum depending on occupation

Operative requirements

- Mini-fragment AO set.
- High arm tourniquet.

Postoperative care

Management

If a strong fixation has been possible, the surgeon may instruct the patient to begin exercising the elbow immediately following surgery. Otherwise an above-elbow back-slab with the elbow at 90° and extending to the metacarpophalangeal joints, is kept on for 2 weeks.

Precise instructions for the physiotherapist should be included in the postoperative instructions within the operation note.

Complications

- Damage to the posterior interosseous nerve leading to a wrist drop.
- Loss of fixation.
- Infection.
- Long-term risk of osteoarthritis.
- Loss of full elbow flexion/extension or supination/pronation.

CHAPTER

23

Arthritis involving the radial head

The condition

Arthritis of the radio-humeral joint occurs commonly in patients with rheumatoid arthritis. Degenerative change may develop secondary to a previous fracture of the radial head.

Making the diagnosis

The patient
The patient usually suffers from widespread rheumatoid arthritis.

The history
The patient complains of pain on pronation and supination, with a restricted range of movement.

On examination
Examine the range of flexion and extension of the elbow, and pronation and supination of the forearm. If the patient only has arthritis affecting the radio-humeral joint, they will only have pain that occurs with pronation and supination. Flexion and extension of the elbow should be pain free.

Feel for crepitus with movement. If the arthritis affects the whole elbow, there may be a flexion contracture and also instability of the collateral ligaments.

Radiographs
AP and lateral views of the elbow are sufficient.

Preoperative management

Investigations

If the patient has rheumatoid arthritis, examine the range of neck and temporo-mandibular movements. Ensure that there is a recent set of cervical spine radiographs to exclude instability.

Treatment

The initial treatment is conservative and includes physiotherapy, splintage to restrict rotation and intra articular steroid injection.

Indications for surgery

Pain originating from the radio-humeral joint that has not responded to conservative treatment.

Operation: excision of the head of the radius

The capsule and part of the annular ligament are divided through a lateral incision centred over the radial head. The neck of the radius is divided, the head removed and the end of the radius smoothed off. Nothing is inserted into the gap created.

Codes

GA/LA	GA
Blood	0
Antibiotics	0
Time	30 minutes
Drains	0
Plaster	Above-elbow back-slab
Postoperative radiograph	0
Stay	Day case
Follow-up	10 days
Off work	2–4 weeks

Operative requirement

High arm tourniquet.

Postoperative care

Management
The arm is rested in an above-elbow plaster back-slab that extends up to the metacarpal heads with the elbow at 90°, for 2 weeks. The patient then gently mobilizes the elbow.

Complications
Injury to the posterior interosseous nerve, resulting in a wrist drop.

24

Arthritis of the elbow

The condition

Severe arthritis of the elbow is common in patients with rheumatoid arthritis. Primary osteoarthritis of the elbow is rare. Secondary osteoarthritis may develop following an intra-articular fracture of the elbow joint.

Making the diagnosis

The patient
The patient usually has polyarticular arthritis involving other upper limb joints.

The history
The most significant symptom is pain. This is usually accompanied by stiffness. Daily activities such as brushing the hair or getting the hand to the mouth may be impossible. You should ask whether the patient can perform 'personal hygiene' after going to the toilet.

On examination
Examine the range of flexion and extension of the elbow, and pronation and supination of the forearm. Feel for crepitus with movement. Note any flexion contracture and/or instability of the collateral ligaments.

Carefully examine the motor and sensory function of the ulnar nerve. If the nerve is compressed, it may need to be transposed during elbow replacement surgery.

Radiographs
AP and lateral views of the elbow are sufficient to show the considerable bony erosion that may have occurred.

Preoperative management

Investigations
If the patient has rheumatoid arthritis, examine the range of neck and temporo-mandibular movements. Ensure that there is a recent set of cervical spine radiographs to exclude instability.

Treatment

Indications for surgery
Once there is severe bony destruction of the joint, that is accompanied by pain, a total elbow replacement can be performed. The aim of the operation is to relieve pain and not to improve the range of movement.

Operation: total elbow replacement (Roper-Tuke)

The elbow is exposed through a posterior midline incision. The end of the humerus is prepared so as to take a metal hemicylindrical prosthesis that is cemented in place. This articulates with a plastic ulnar component that sits in the coronoid fossa and is held with a screw that passes down the shaft of the ulna.

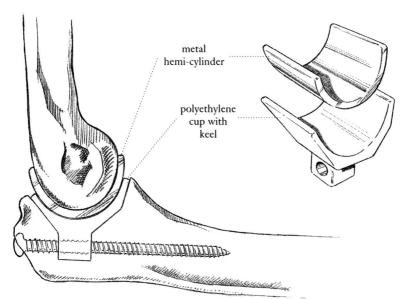

metal
hemi-cylinder

polyethylene
cup with
keel

Codes

GA/LA	GA
Blood	Group and save
Antibiotics	Yes
Time	1.5 hours
Drains	Yes
Plaster	Above elbow
Postoperative radiograph	AP and lateral elbow
Stay	3 or 4 days
Follow-up	Readmit after 3 weeks for inpatient physiotherapy
Off work	3 months

Operative requirement
High arm tourniquet.

Postoperative care

Management
Check that the ulnar nerve is intact by testing sensation in the ulnar one and a half fingers and the power of finger abduction.

The elbow is rested in a back-slab for 3 weeks, after which time it is gently mobilized.

Complications
- Ulnar nerve dysfunction.
- Instability of the elbow.
- Loosening.
- Infection.
- Dislocation.

25

CHAPTER

Compression of the ulnar nerve at the elbow

The condition

The ulnar nerve can be compressed as it passes through the cubital tunnel. Sensory symptoms usually precede motor symptoms.

Making the diagnosis

The history

The patient complains of numbness in the ulnar nerve distribution and of weakness in the hand. Typically the patient wakes at night complaining of numbness. There may be a history of previous bony trauma, commonly a supra-condylar fracture of the humerus that has resulted in a valgus elbow.

On examination

Examine the alignment and range of movement of the elbow.

Examine the ulnar nerve sensory and motor function of both arms; i.e. sensation in the ulnar one and a half fingers, power in the long flexor to the little finger and power of abductor digiti minimi. Ask the patient to hold their elbow fully flexed for 1 minute and see if this brings on their numbness. Note how long it takes for the numbness to appear.

In severe cases there may be wasting of the first dorsal interosseous muscle or even an ulnar claw hand.

Investigations

An electromyogram will establish the site and nature of the lesion.

Radiographs

AP and lateral views of the elbow.

Treatment

The initial treatment should be conservative. Many patients' symptoms will improve with the use of a night-splint that keeps the elbow extended. The splint may have to be worn every night for 6 months.

Indications for surgery

Persistent symptoms of ulnar nerve dysfunction confirmed by an abnormal electromyogram and failure of conservative treatment.

Operation: decompression ± transposition of the ulnar nerve

The nerve is exposed through an incision made directly over it. The commonly performed procedures are:

1. Simple decompression of the nerve in the cubital tunnel without transposition.

2. Anterior subcutaneous transposition.

3. Anterior submuscular transposition, with the nerve being placed under the flexor muscles. This submuscular anterior transposition has the longest recovery period.

Codes

GA/LA	GA
Blood	0
Antibiotics	0
Time	1 hour
Drains	0
Plaster	Above elbow
Postoperative radiograph	0
Stay	Day case
Follow-up	10 days
Off work	3 weeks

Operative requirement

High arm tourniquet.

Postoperative care

Management
Check the motor and sensory function of the ulnar nerve.

The arm is immobilized by an above-elbow back-slab for 2 weeks prior to gentle active mobilization.

Complications
Temporary or permanent worsening of the ulnar nerve dysfunction.

CHAPTER

26

Olecranon bursitis

The condition

The olecranon bursa may become inflamed as a result of friction or pressure. Other uncommon causes include gout, in which the lump may be calcified, or rheumatoid arthritis.

Making the diagnosis

The history
The patient complains of recurrent swelling and pain at the tip of the elbow. The bursa may become secondarily infected.

On examination
The bursa is over the very point of the elbow. If it has been inflamed but is not acutely inflamed when you examine the patient, it may be looser and more sack-like than normal, with a thickened wall.

Radiographs
A lateral radiograph of the elbow may show calcification within the bursa.

Treatment

Most episodes of inflammation can be managed conservatively with a combination of an oral non-steroidal anti-inflammatory drug, aspiration of the bursa and injection of steroid into the bursa.

Indications for surgery
Recurrent bursitis that has not responded to conservative treatment.

Operation: excision of the olecranon bursa

The bursa is completely excised through a longitudinal posterior incision.

Codes

GA/LA	GA
Blood	0
Antibiotics	Optional
Time	30 minutes
Drains	Sometimes
Plaster	0
Postoperative radiograph	0
Stay	1 night
Follow-up	10 days
Off work	3 weeks

Operative requirement
Tourniquet.

Postoperative care

Management
The dressings are reduced and the drain is removed after 24 hours. Immediate mobilization of the elbow is encouraged, but the elbow can be rested in a sling between times.

Complications
- Wound infection.
- Wound haematoma.
- Injury to the ulnar nerve.

CHAPTER 27

Fracture of the shafts of the radius and ulna

The condition

When both bones of the forearm are fractured, they may be either displaced or undisplaced. If a single bone is broken and is displaced, there *must* be another discontinuity in the rectangle formed by the radius, the ulna, and the proximal and distal radio-ulnar joints. A Monteggia fracture is the combination of a proximal ulnar fracture with dislocation of the radial head at the elbow. A Galeazzi fracture is a fracture of the distal radius with dislocation of the distal ulna.

Making the diagnosis

The patient
This injury can occur in a patient of any age.

On examination
The diagnosis is usually clinically obvious. Examine the neuro-vascular integrity of the hand. If there is restriction in extension of the fingers or abnormal sensation in the fingers, the patient may be developing a compartment syndrome. An urgent fasciotomy may be necessary.

Note the presence and location of any grazes or fracture blisters, as these may prevent immediate open reduction.

Radiographs
Order AP and lateral views of the whole forearm including the wrist and elbow. Look for dislocation of the radial head at the elbow or the ulna at the wrist.

Preoperative management

Common associated injuries
Compartment syndrome.
Injury to the nerves or vessels of the forearm.

Preparation for surgery
Rest and immobilize the arm in a well-padded above-elbow back-slab.

Treatment

Indications for surgery
In children, some angulation on the lateral radiograph is acceptable. The younger the patient, the greater the potential for remodelling with growth and therefore the greater the angulation that can be accepted.

Varus or valgus deformity, or rotational deformity will not remodel with growth and therefore must be corrected.

In adults, only completely undisplaced fractures of both bones are treated conservatively in a plaster. Even then careful follow-up with radiographs after 1, 2 and 3 weeks is mandatory. If the fracture displaces it should be internally fixed. All displaced fractures in an adult require open reduction and internal fixation.

Operation: manipulation under anaesthesia of fractured radius and ulna in a child

The fracture is manipulated under a general anaesthetic and the position checked with the image intensifier. The limb is then immobilized in a well-padded above-elbow back-slab, or a full plaster that is split.

Codes
GA/LA	GA
Blood	0
Antibiotics	0
Time	30 minutes
Drains	0
Plaster	Above elbow
Postoperative radiograph	AP and lateral radius and ulna

Stay   1 night
Follow-up   1 week, X-ray on arrival
Off school   1 week

Operative requirements
Image intensifier and radiographer.

Postoperative care

Management
Elevate the arm on pillows. Instruct the nurses to carefully monitor the neuro-vascular status of the hand. Beware compartment syndrome! An immobilized, reduced fracture should not be very painful. If the child is in a lot of pain, do not just increase the analgesics, but go and see the patient. Split the plaster and padding down to the skin. If you are concerned, call the surgeon whatever the time of day!

Complications
- Compartment syndrome.
- Loss of position.
- Malunion.
- Restricted pronation or supination due to persistent rotational malunion.

Operation: open reduction and internal fixation of the radius and ulna in an adult

The ulna is exposed through an incision over the subcutaneous border of the bone. The radius is approached through either an anterior or a lateral incision. The vital structures such as the radial artery and radial nerve have to be seen and protected as part of the anterior exposure of the radius. The fractures are reduced and then held using plates and screws.

Codes
GA/LA   GA
Blood   0
Antibiotics   Yes
Time   1.5 hours

Drains	Yes
Plaster	0
Postoperative radiograph	AP and lateral radius and ulna
Stay	3 days
Follow-up	10 days
Off work	4 weeks

Operative requirements

- Small fragment AO set.
- High arm tourniquet.

Postoperative care

Management

- Elevate the arm on two pillows.
- Carefully monitor the neuro-vascular function in the hand.
- Beware compartment syndrome.
- Encourage the patient to mobilize the hand and elbow.

Complications

- Compartment syndrome.
- Neurapraxia or division of the radial, ulnar or median nerve.
- Infection.
- Non-union.
- Late fracture of the forearm at the plate/non-plate junction.

CHAPTER **28**

Removal of internal fixation of the forearm

The condition

After a forearm fracture that was fixed using plates and screws has united, one can remove the metal work.

The argument for removing the metal work is that there is an increased risk of fracture of the bone at the point where the plate ends. This is because the plate is a stress riser. In other words, due to the plate's rigidity, the force of the fall is concentrated at one point. Fixation of these fractures is difficult.

The argument against removing the plates, is that surgery is associated with a real risk of nerve injury that is greater than the original operation. This is because scar tissue makes identification of vital structures difficult.

Treatment

Indications for surgery

A healed forearm fracture, at least 18 months following internal fixation, in a patient less than 40 years. If a patient complains that they can feel the ulnar plate under the skin, some surgeons just remove the plate from the ulna. The radial plate may be left in situ.

Operation: removal of plates from radius and ulna

The plates are exposed and removed through the original incisions.

Codes
GA/LA	GA
Blood	0
Antibiotics	0
Time	45 minutes

104

Drains	Yes
Plaster	0
Postoperative radiograph	AP and lateral forearm
Stay	2 days
Follow-up	10 days
Off work	3 weeks

Operative requirements
- Tourniquet.
- Screwdriver of the appropriate size and type. This will probably be the screwdriver for AO small fragment screws.

Postoperative care

Management
The arm does not need to be immobilized.

The patient must be aware that following the removal of the plates, the bones can fracture with less force than is required to break a normal bone. This is because the bone that was under the plates has been shielded from stress and is thus weaker than normal. It takes 3–6 months for the bones to regain normal strength. The patient can use the arm for normal activities immediately postoperatively, but should do no sport for 3 months and avoid extreme activities for 6 months.

Complications
The incidence of complications following removal of plates is much higher than following their insertion:
- Nerve injury.
- Wound infection.
- Unsightly scar.
- Refracture.

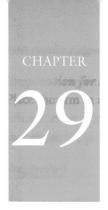

CHAPTER 29

Fracture/separation of the epiphysis of the distal radius

The condition

This is the equivalent in children to a Colles' fracture in an adult.

Making the diagnosis

The patient
A child between 8 years old and their teens.

The history
The history will be of a fall onto the outstretched hand. The child will complain of a painful wrist.

On examination
The wrist is swollen, painful and may be deformed. Gently examine the whole forearm and elbow to exclude a more proximal injury.

Radiographs
Obtain AP and lateral views of the wrist. If only one bone is fractured at the wrist, there may be a fracture more proximally. Beware missing a Galeazzi combination of a fractured radius with dislocation of the distal radio-ulnar joint. If in doubt, X-ray the whole forearm and also the uninjured side for comparison.

Preoperative management

Preparation for surgery
Rest the wrist in a well-padded below-elbow back-slab.

106

Treatment

The younger the child, the greater the potential for remodelling with growth of a displaced fracture. If the displacement is minimal, the added trauma of a manipulation may not be necessary and may further injure the growth plate.

Indications for surgery
A fracture that is significantly displaced.

Operation: manipulation under anaesthesia of a fractured distal radius in a child with or without K-wire insertion

The wrist is gently manipulated. Flexion of the fracture is usually the only manoeuvre necessary for a slightly displaced fracture. The reduction is checked with the image intensifier and a plaster cast is applied which is immediately split. If the fracture is significantly displaced, it may be potentially unstable after it has been reduced. In these cases it is best to stabilize the radius with one or two K-wires. They are inserted through stab incisions in the skin. They are left protruding so they can easily be removed in the outpatient department. A cast is applied after the wires have been inserted.

Codes
GA/LA	GA
Blood	0
Antibiotics	0
Time	30 minutes
Drains	0
Plaster	Below elbow
Postoperative radiograph	AP and lateral wrist
Stay	1 night
Follow-up	1 week, X-ray on arrival
Off school	1 week

Operative requirements
- Image intensifier and radiographer.
- K-wire set.

Postoperative care

Management

Elevate the arm and encourage early finger movement.

Carefully monitor the neuro-vascular status of the hand. Beware compartment syndrome!

The length of time that the cast is kept on depends on the age of the child. In young children, 3 weeks is adequate. In teenagers, 6 weeks is necessary.

If a K-wire is inserted it is removed after 3 weeks. It is usually removed in the outpatient department with minimal discomfort.

Complications

- Compartment syndrome.
- Loss of position.
- Abnormal growth.

CHAPTER 30

Colles' fracture

The condition

A Colles' fracture is defined as a fracture of the distal radius that is 2.5 cm (1 inch) from the wrist joint, with the distal fragment being dorsally tilted, impacted, and often radially displaced (originally described in 1814 by Abraham Colles).

Making the diagnosis

The patient
Typically a postmenopausal woman.

The history
A fall onto an outstretched hand resulting in a painful wrist.

On examination
The wrist is usually swollen. If the fracture is grossly displaced, there is a 'dinner fork' deformity.

Examine the neuro-vascular status of the hand. Acute carpal tunnel syndrome can occur, resulting in paraesthesia in the radial three and a half fingers.

Radiographs
Order AP and lateral radiographs of the wrist. Ensure that the orientation is correct when you are looking at the lateral view: with the forearm horizontal and the thumb pointing down, the distal fragment will be tipped up and back if it is a Colles' fracture. If it is tipped down, you are looking at a Smith's fracture.

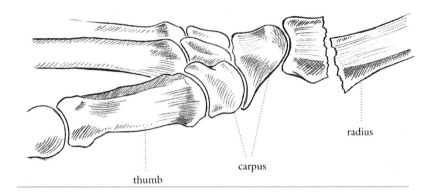

radius

carpus

thumb

Ensure that the crescentic outline of the lunate is in line with the radius and in line with capitate. If it is not, it may be dislocated downwards and pressing on the median nerve!

Preoperative management

Common associated injuries
Other fractures associated with osteoporosis, in particular the neck of the femur.

Preparation for surgery
Rest the wrist in a back-slab.

Treatment

If the fracture is undisplaced or minimally displaced, the wrist is simply immobilized in a below-elbow cast.

If the fracture is displaced, it may need to be reduced. The amount of displacement that is acceptable, increases with the age of the patient. In a 40-year-old, no displacement is acceptable. In a 90-year-old, considerable displacement is accepted.

If the fracture is not comminuted, manipulation and application of a cast is usually sufficient.

If the fracture has a lot of dorsal comminution, so it is likely to redisplace, the reduction can be held with percutaneous K-wires.

If the whole fracture is comminuted, the radius can be held out to length using an external fixator. Sometimes it is necessary to insert K-wires *and* apply an external fixator.

Indications for surgery
A fracture that is significantly displaced.
A fracture that was previously manipulated and has lost its position.

Operation: manipulation under anaesthesia of Colles' fracture ± application of external fixator ± insertion of K-wires

When manipulating a Colles' fracture, the aim is to:
1. Restore the radius to its proper length in relation to the ulna on the AP view of the wrist.
2. Restore the angle of the articular surface of the radius to 15° of palmar flexion.

If an external fixator is used to hold the reduction, two pins are inserted into the second (index) metacarpal and two into the radius, proximal to the fracture.

K-wires are inserted through small stab incisions and the ends are left protruding so that they can easily be removed. A wire can be passed through the fracture on one cortex and then into the intact bone of the far proximal cortex. It then acts as a buttress. This is the Kapandji technique (see below).

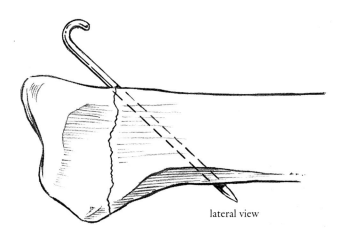

lateral view

Codes

GA/LA	GA or regional block
Blood	0
Antibiotics	0
Time	30 minutes
Drains	0
Plaster	Below elbow, unless external fixator applied
Postoperative radiograph	AP and lateral wrist
Stay	24 hours
Follow-up	1 week, X-ray on arrival
Off work	2–6 weeks depending on occupation

Operative requirements

- Image intensifier.
- K-wire set.
- Small external fixator.

Postoperative care

Management

Elevate the hand for 24 hours. Encourage the patient to mobilize the fingers, elbow and shoulder once they go home. A sling, if used, should be discarded after 24 hours.

If the wrist is in a cast, the fracture may redisplace up to 2 weeks following reduction. Therefore, the patient must be seen in the fracture clinic and the position checked with a radiograph after 1 and after 2 weeks.

The wrist is kept in a cast for 3–6 weeks.

If the fracture has been held with K-wires, these are removed in the outpatient department after 3–4 weeks and the wrist is immobilized in a plaster cast for a further 2 weeks.

If the fracture has been stabilized with an external fixator, this is removed in the outpatient department after 6 weeks.

Complications

- Loss of position. This can occur up to 2 weeks after manipulation of the fracture.
- Pin track infection leading to early removal of the external fixator.
- Carpal tunnel syndrome.
- Late Dupuytren's contracture.

31 Intra-articular fracture of the distal radius

The condition

These fractures are more difficult to treat than a simple Colles' fracture. If the joint surface is not restored to near normal, the patient may have a poor result.

Making the diagnosis

The patient
Young and middle-aged adults.

The history
A fall onto an outstretched hand resulting in a painful wrist.

Considerable force is required to sustain these severe fractures in strong healthy bone. Less force is required in osteoporotic bone.

On examination
The wrist is usually swollen.

Examine the neuro-vascular status of the hand. Acute carpal tunnel syndrome can occur, resulting in paraesthesia in the radial three and a half fingers.

Radiographs
Order AP and lateral radiographs of the wrist. Ensure that the orientation is correct when you are looking at the lateral view.

Look at the distal radius carefully. Are there multiple fragments or just two or three? How short is the radius relative to the ulna?

If the configuration of the fracture is not clear on plain radiographs, order tomograms or a CT scan of the wrist.

Preoperative management

Preparation for surgery

If the wrist is grossly displaced and definitive treatment is likely to be delayed by a more than a few hours, perform a manipulation in the casualty. This may be done using a haematoma block or regional block since you are not aiming for a perfect reduction. This will reduce the patient's pain, allow to you to obtain further radiographs or other scans, and reduce the risk of median nerve compression.

Rest the wrist in a back-slab.

Treatment

Treatment of these fractures is challenging. If the bone is of normal quality, one can perform an open reduction and internal fixation with or without bone grafting. If the bone is osteoporotic, the radius can be held out to length using an external fixator. Sometimes it is necessary to insert K-wires, apply an external fixator and insert bone graft through a limited dorsal incision.

Indications for surgery

- A fracture that is significantly displaced.
- A fracture that was previously manipulated and has lost its position.

The aim of surgery is to restore the joint surface of the distal radius to as near normal as possible. Once reduced the fracture fragments have to be held in place while the fracture unites.

The final decision as to the best method of treatment is often not possible until the fracture has been manipulated in theatre and examined under the image intensifier.

Operation: manipulation under anaesthesia of distal radius fracture ± application of external fixator ± insertion of K-wires ± bone grafting

If an external fixator is used to hold the reduction, two pins are inserted into the second (index) metacarpal and two into the radius, proximal to the fracture.

K-wires are inserted through small stab incisions and the ends are left protruding so that they can be removed easily.

If the lunate fossa of the radius is depressed, it can be elevated by pushing a blunt instrument in through a small incision on the dorsum of the wrist. Similar to a tibial plateau fracture, bone graft is then used to fill the void that occurs by elevating the fracture fragment.

Bone graft is usually taken from the iliac crest. If there is any possibility of bone graft being required, you must include this on the consent.

Operation: open reduction and internal fixation of distal radius fracture ± bone grafting

If the fracture fragments are displaced dorsally, we make a straight dorsal incision. The fracture is reduced under direct vision. A plate is applied to the dorsal surface of the radius. This is not as easy as it may seem due to the presence of the extensor tendons and the extensor retinaculum.

If the fracture fragments are displaced palmarwards, the approach is the same as for a simple Smith's fracture. The fracture is exposed through a longitudinal incision on the front of the wrist. The dissection is through the interval between the flexor carpi radialis tendon and the flexor tendons, or between the flexor carpi radialis tendon and the radial artery. The fracture is reduced and then the distal fragments are held in position with a 'T' plate that acts as a buttress.

Codes

GA/LA	GA
Blood	0
Antibiotics	0
Time	1 hour
Drains	0
Plaster	Below elbow, unless external fixator applied
Postoperative radiograph	AP and lateral wrist
Stay	24 hours
Follow-up	1 week, X-ray on arrival
Off work	2–6 weeks depending on occupation

Operative requirements

- Image intensifier.
- K-wire set.
- Small external fixator.
- Small fragment AO set.

Postoperative care

Management

Elevate the hand for 24 hours. Encourage the patient to mobilize the fingers, elbow and shoulder once they go home. A sling, if used, should be discarded after 24 hours.

If the wrist is in a cast, the fracture may redisplace up to 2 weeks following reduction. Therefore, the patient must be seen in the fracture clinic and the position checked with a radiograph after 1 and after 2 weeks.

If the fracture has been held with K-wires, these are removed in the outpatient department after 3–4 weeks and the wrist is immobilized in a plaster cast for a further 2 weeks.

If the fracture has been stabilized with an external fixator, this is removed in the outpatient department after 6 weeks.

Complications

- Pin track infection leading to early removal of the external fixator.
- Carpal tunnel syndrome.
- Late Dupuytren's contracture.
- Loss of some flexion and extension, and/or pronation and supination.

CHAPTER

32

Smith's fracture

The condition

A fracture of the distal radius that is 2.5 cm (1 inch) from the wrist joint, with the distal fragment being tilted towards the palm (described by R. W. Smith in 1847).

Making the diagnosis

The patient
Typically a postmenopausal woman.

The history
A fall onto the back of the hand.

On examination
The wrist is deformed.

Examine the neuro-vascular status of the hand as an acute carpal tunnel syndrome is common, with resultant paraesthesia in the radial three and a half fingers.

Radiographs
Request AP and lateral radiographs of the wrist. When looking at the lateral view, ensure that the orientation is correct, i.e. with the thumb pointing down. In this position the distal fragment will be tipped down. If it is tipped up, it is a Colles' fracture.

Preoperative management

Common associated injuries
Other fractures associated with osteoporosis, in particular a fracture of the neck of the femur.

Preparation for surgery
Rest the wrist in a back-slab.

Treatment

Any fracture that is displaced needs to be reduced. Initially a closed manipulation can be performed. However, loss of position is common and the fracture then requires open reduction and internal fixation.

Indications for surgery
Open reduction and internal fixation is required if the fracture cannot be manipulated into a satisfactory position or if a good reduction has been lost.

Operation: open reduction and internal fixation of Smith's fracture

The fracture is exposed through a longitudinal incision on the front of the wrist. The dissection is through the interval between the flexor carpi radialis tendon and the flexor tendons, or between the flexor carpi radialis tendon and the radial artery. The fracture is reduced and then the distal fragment is held in position with a 'T' plate that acts as a buttress. The plate is only screwed to the proximal fragment, since the distal fragment is usually too porotic to hold screws.

Codes

GA/LA	GA
Blood	0
Antibiotics	Yes
Time	1 hour
Drains	0
Plaster	Below elbow, 2–3 weeks
Postoperative radiograph	AP and lateral wrist
Stay	2 days
Follow-up	10 days
Off work	2–6 weeks depending on occupation

Operative requirements
- Small fragment AO set.
- Plain films or image intensifier plus radiographer.

Postoperative care

Management

Elevate the hand and encourage finger, elbow and shoulder movement. If used, discard the sling after 24 hours. (The plate is not removed once the fracture has united.)

Complications

- Loss of position.
- Acute carpal tunnel syndrome.

33 Painful distal radio-ulnar joint

The condition

A patient may have pain around the distal radio-ulnar joint due to malunion of a previous wrist fracture, or due to rheumatoid arthritis.

Making the diagnosis

The history

The patient may have had a fractured wrist previously. They often comment that the ulna became more prominent following the fracture. Alternatively the patient may have rheumatoid arthritis.

The patient may complain of pain around the distal ulna that is made worse by activities that involve twisting the wrist, for example using a door handle, opening a door with a key or unscrewing the top off a jar.

On examination

The distal ulna may be very prominent. Hold the patient's elbow at 90° and examine their range of pronation and supination. Gently feel for crepitus as they twist the wrist from palm up (supinated) to palm down (pronated).

Examine the motor and sensory function of the ulnar nerve in the hand. Check the integrity of the extensor tendons.

Radiographs

AP and lateral views of the wrist are adequate.

Preoperative management

Preparation for surgery

If the patient suffers from rheumatoid arthritis, examine their neck movements and check that they can open their mouth wide. Ensure that there is a recent set of radiographs of the cervical spine if they have any neck symptoms.

Treatment

Indications for surgery

There is little conservative treatment other than anti-inflammatory medication for this problem. Surgery is indicated if the pain is severe and limits the patient's hand function.

In young adults one can preserve support to the ulnar side of the wrist. We fuse the distal radio-ulnar joint and excise a piece of ulna more proximally to allow pronation and supination.

In older patients and in those with rheumatoid arthritis, excision of the distal ulna is a reliable and benign procedure.

Operation: excision of the distal ulna (Darrach procedure)

We make an incision along the ulnar border of the wrist. We remove the distal 2 cm of the ulna using a powered saw.

Codes

GA/LA	GA or Biers
Blood	0
Antibiotics	0
Time	30 minutes
Drains	Sometimes
Plaster	0
Postoperative radiograph	0
Stay	Day case
Follow-up	10 days
Off work	2 weeks

Operative requirements
- Small powered saw.
- Tourniquet.

Postoperative care

Management
Encourage the patient to use their arm and hand as the pain settles.

Complications
Injury to the ulnar nerve, usually a neurapraxia rather than a permanent injury.

Operation: Sauve-Kapandji procedure (distal radio-ulnar fusion with proximal pseudarthrosis)

We make a 8 cm incision along the ulnar border of the wrist. We then remove a segment of the ulna proximal to the distal radioulnar joint. We fuse the radioulnar joint and fix the ulna to the radius with a screw and/or a K-wire. The aim is to allow pronation and supination to occur at the ulnar pseudarthrosis.

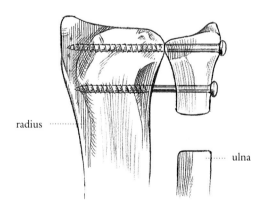

Codes

GA/LA	GA
Blood	0
Antibiotics	Yes

Time	1.5 hours
Drains	Sometimes
Plaster	Below elbow
Postoperative radiograph	AP and lateral wrist
Stay	1 night
Follow-up	10 days
Off work	2 weeks

Operative requirements
■ Small power saw, small fragment screws or small cannulated screws.
■ Tourniquet.
■ Image intensifier.

Postoperative care

Management
■ Elevate the arm for the first 24 hours.
■ Encourage the patient to move their fingers.

Complications
■ Failure of the ulnar styloid to fuse to the radius.
■ Ossification of the ulnar pseudarthrosis restricting pronation and supination.

Carpal tunnel syndrome

The condition

The median nerve is compressed as it passes through the carpal canal at the wrist.

Making the diagnosis

The patient

The syndrome is common in postmenopausal women, in pregnancy, in rheumatoid arthritis and following a wrist fracture. However, in 50% of the patients, no predisposing cause is found.

The history

The patient complains of pain and tingling in the fingers. This may involve all the fingers, but typically affects only the radial three and a half digits, with sparing of the little finger. The symptoms are often worse at night, with the patient waking with a numb hand that they shake 'trying to restore the circulation'.

The patient may complain of an inability to pick up a fine object such as a pin.

Many patients complain of discomfort or pain that radiates up to or even beyond the elbow.

On examination

Examine the light touch sensation in each finger, on each half of the palmar side.

Test the power of thumb abduction.

Percuss over the median nerve at the wrist to elicit Tinel's sign. This is positive if percussion over the nerve generates paraesthesia (tingling) in the fingers.

Phalen's test is the most reliable clinical test for carpal tunnel syndrome. It is performed by holding the patient's forearm vertically and allowing their wrist and hand to fall into palmar-flexion. This may reproduce the patient's symptoms within 1 minute. It is best to time the test. It is more significant if the patient complains of tingling after 10 seconds than after 1 minute.

Radiographs
AP and lateral radiographs of the wrist are necessary to exclude a bony cause for the nerve compression.

Preoperative management

Investigations
The diagnosis should be confirmed with an electromyogram if surgery is contemplated.

Treatment

If symptoms have commenced during pregnancy, they usually resolve after delivery. In patients with mild symptoms, a wrist splint (Futura splint), worn at night, may be helpful.

If the electromyogram does not show slowing of conduction in the motor component of the median nerve, a local steroid injection around the nerve at the wrist may alleviate the symptoms. Steroid injection usually relieves symptoms for a few months. The symptoms then usually recur.

Surgery reliably relieves the symptoms in patients with established median nerve compression. Most surgeons perform a open decompression under local anaesthetic.

Some centres perform surgery using a small arthroscope and a special knife introduced through two small incisions. The complication rate for this 'keyhole' technique is high, especially when gaining experience. As a result the technique is not widely performed.

Indications for surgery
Carpal tunnel syndrome, preferably proven with an electromyogram.

Operation: decompression of the carpal canal

We make an incision in the palm parallel to the thenar skin crease. We divide the transverse carpal ligament under direct vision. We keep the incision through the ligament towards the ulnar side of the median nerve. This is to reduce the risk of injury to the motor branch to the thumb.

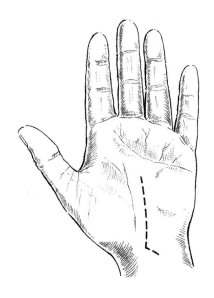

Codes

GA/LA	LA or GA
Blood	0
Antibiotics	0
Time	30 minutes
Drains	0
Plaster	0
Postoperative radiograph	0
Stay	Day case
Follow-up	10 days
Off work	2 weeks

Operative requirement

High arm tourniquet.

Postoperative care

Management
- Elevate the arm on two pillows.
- Check the integrity of thumb abduction before the patient is discharged.

Complications
- Division of the motor nerve to the thumb.
- Division of the palmar cutaneous nerve.
- A feeling of weakness of grip that takes several months to settle.
- Recurrence of median nerve compression.

35

Wrist ganglion

The condition

A ganglion is a cyst containing viscous fluid. It can occur anywhere in the hand. It is usually in continuity with a joint or tendon sheath. The lump may alter in size and although not in itself tender, it may be associated with some pain around the wrist.

Making the diagnosis

The patient
Usually a young adult. Ganglions can occur in children. Ganglions are uncommon in the elderly.

The history
The ganglion is normally on the dorsum of the wrist. It may vary in size over a period of weeks or months. There may be some aching on use of the wrist. Always ask if there has been any previous trauma to the wrist.

On examination
The lump is firm and not fixed to the skin but it may be fixed to the underlying structures. It is usually on the dorsum of the wrist but may be on the palmar aspect.

Radiographs
Always obtain AP and lateral radiographs of the wrist to exclude bony pathology and to see if there are any degenerative changes in the wrist or carpal joints. If there is any doubt about the diagnosis, the best investigation is an ultrasound.

Treatment

A ganglion can be aspirated. This is done in the clinic and has a high cure rate. It is simple to do and if successful saves the patient an operation and a scar.

Indications for surgery

A ganglion that has recurred after aspiration. The patient must accept that ganglions may recur after excision and that they will have a scar.

Contra-indications to surgery

A patient who is unwilling to exchange a lump for a scar. Therefore always ensure that the patient is aware that they will have a scar that will be at least as long as the diameter of the lump and that the operation site will be quite painful for some time.

Operation: excision of wrist ganglion

The ganglion is freed from the surrounding tissue and followed down to its base. Ideally this is done without bursting the ganglion. The ganglion is then excised.

Codes

GA/LA	LA or regional
Blood	0
Antibiotics	0
Time	30 minutes
Drains	0
Plaster	0
Postoperative radiograph	0
Stay	Day case
Follow-up	10 days
Off work	10 days

Operative requirement
Tourniquet.

Postoperative care

Management
Elevate the hand for the first day postoperatively.

Complications
There is a real risk of recurrence after excision that is at least 30%. Alternatively, a new ganglion may develop close to the site of the previous one.

Removal of ganglions on the dorsum of the wrist has minimal additional complications. Ganglions on the palmar aspect have a risk of adjacent vital structures being damaged when the ganglion is excised. Also, the preoperative diagnosis may have been incorrect and the mass may, for example, be a tumour of the median nerve, which should not be excised by the inexperienced.

Fractured scaphoid

The condition

The scaphoid is the most frequently fractured carpal bone. It can be difficult to diagnose the fracture with certainty. Even if a fracture is diagnosed and correctly treated, a scaphoid fracture may fail to unite.

Making the diagnosis

The patient
Scaphoid fractures are rare in the skeletally immature (prior to closure of the epiphyses) and unusual after middle age.

The history
The patient usually recalls falling onto his outstretched hand. He will complain of wrist pain, especially at the base of the thumb.

On examination
The signs of a scaphoid fracture include pain in the anatomical snuff box, pain over the pole of the scaphoid (felt in the base of the thenar eminence), pain on distraction of the thumb and pain on compression along the thumb. Only one of these signs may be present.

Always palpate the 'normal' anatomical snuff box, as the terminal branch of the superficial nerve lies in the base and pressing on the nerve may be painful. Then compare the normal with the abnormal.

Radiographs
Always request AP and lateral views of the wrist, and 'scaphoid views'. If the scaphoid appears clinically fractured, but the radiographs

are normal, it is traditional to repeat the radiographs after 10 days, when the fracture may be more easily seen. This is because the bone at the fracture resorbs a little.

If there is doubt about the diagnosis, you should order a radio-isotope bone scan. This will show a 'hot spot' over the scaphoid if it is fractured.

Treatment

The majority of scaphoid fractures that are proven clinically and radio-logically, are successfully treated in a below-elbow plaster cast. The traditional scaphoid cast extends up to the inter-phalangeal joint of the thumb, with the hand positioned as if holding a wine glass. However it has been proven that the rate of union is unchanged if a simple below-elbow cast is used that extends only to the metacarpophalangeal joint of the thumb. This type of cast allows the patient much greater hand function.

Immobilization needs to be continued until the fracture has united. This may take up to 3 months.

Indications for surgery
If the scaphoid fracture is displaced, it is unlikely to unite. A displaced fracture should be internally fixed acutely. Bone grafting is not needed.

If an undisplaced fracture fails to unite after conservative treatment the scaphoid needs open reduction, bone grafting and internal fixation with a compression screw.

Operation: internal fixation and bone grafting of non-union of a scaphoid fracture with a Herbert-Whipple screw

The scaphoid is exposed through an incision that crosses the wrist on the flexor aspect. Bone graft is either taken locally from the distal radius or from the iliac crest and packed into the fracture.

The Herbert-Whipple screw is cannulated (unlike the Herbert screw). There is a special jig to align the drill. Its main design features are the lack of a head and the differential pitch of the threads at each end, which gives compression of the fracture as the screw is tightened.

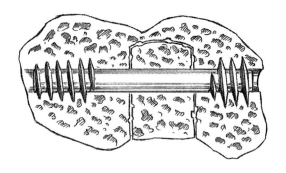

Codes

GA/LA	GA
Blood	0
Antibiotics	Yes
Time	1 hour
Drains	0
Plaster	Below elbow
Postoperative radiograph	Scaphoid views
Stay	1 night
Follow-up	10 days
Off work	2 weeks

Operative requirements

- High-arm tourniquet.
- Herbert screw set.
- Image intensifier and radiographer.

Postoperative care

Management

Check the postoperative radiographs to ensure that the screw does not protrude out of the proximal pole of the scaphoid into the wrist joint.

The cast is usually retained for 4–6 weeks and then the patient is allowed to mobilize the wrist.

Complications

- Comminution of the fracture.
- Persistent non-union.

37 Trigger finger

The condition

Trigger finger occurs as a result of a nodule forming on the flexor tendon just before the most proximal pulley of the tendon sheath. When the digit is flexed, the nodule comes out of the tendon sheath. The nodule then prevents the tendon gliding smoothly back into the tendon sheath when the patient tries to extend the finger. Sometimes the nodule suddenly pops into the tendon sheath allowing the finger to suddenly extend. Hence the name trigger finger.

Making the diagnosis

The patient

Trigger thumb may occur in babies and toddlers. It is sometimes called congenital trigger thumb although most are not abnormal at birth.

Triggering is common in adults in middle age and beyond. It may occur in patients with rheumatoid arthritis, but most patients have no obvious predisposing condition. The ring and middle fingers are most commonly affected.

The history

Babies with trigger thumb are brought by their parents with the history that the thumb will not straighten.

Adults may complain of pain around the base of the finger and often state that the finger can only be straightened by using the other hand, or by using the adjacent finger. The patient may mistakenly feel that the problem is located around the proximal interphalangeal joint.

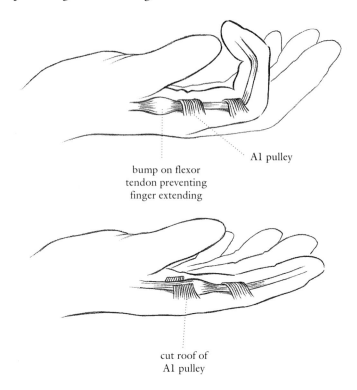

bump on flexor
tendon preventing
finger extending

A1 pulley

cut roof of
A1 pulley

On examination

Many patients can produce the triggering for you to see. There is usually a lump on the flexor tendon just proximal to the metacarpal head, which may be tender.

Treatment

Trigger finger in adults is often cured by an injection of local steroid around the entrance to the flexor canal. This is done in outpatients.

Prepare a syringe containing 1 ml of 1% lignocaine mixed with 1 ml of depot steroid (e.g. depomedrone or lederspan). Use a fine gauge needle. Feel for the bump on the flexor tendon as the patient flexes and extends the finger. Prepare the injection site by cleaning the skin with alcohol. Let the alcohol dry before inserting the needle. Advance the needle towards the flexor tendons. Ask the patient to gently move the finger. If your needle moves it is in the tendon and you must withdraw it a little. If the needle does not move with the tendon, advance until you feel the tendon scraping along the needle. Inject 1 ml of the anaesthetic steroid mixture. The injection must go in with ease. If it does not you may be trying to inject into the tendon which will damage the tendon.

Indications for surgery

Trigger thumb can resolve spontaneously in babies. However if the thumb stays permanently flexed for many months many surgeons will not wait too long before operating.

In adults conservative treatment with steroid injection should be tried. If the triggering recurs after two injections, surgery is required.

Operation: release of trigger thumb in a baby

The first annular (A1) pulley, which forms the entrance to the flexor sheath, is divided through a transverse or longitudinal incision at the base of the thumb. The tendon itself needs no treatment.

Codes

GA/LA	GA
Blood	0
Antibiotics	0
Time	20 minutes
Drains	0
Plaster	0
Postoperative radiograph	0
Stay	Day case
Follow-up	10 days

Operative requirement

Paediatric tourniquet.

Postoperative care

Management

Babies do not need physiotherapy and they will start to use the thumb after the discomfort from the operation has settled.

Complications

Division of a digital nerve to the thumb.

Operation: release of trigger finger in an adult

The first annular (A1) pulley, which forms the entrance to the flexor sheath, is divided through a 1 cm transverse incision, just beyond the distal palmar crease. If performed under LA the patient should be able to flex and extend the digit while the wound is open and demonstrate that it no longer triggers.

Codes

GA/LA	LA
Blood	0
Antibiotics	0
Time	20 minutes
Drains	0
Plaster	0
Postoperative radiograph	0
Stay	Day case
Follow-up	10 days
Off work	Depends on occupation

Operative requirement
Tourniquet.

Postoperative care

Management
Encourage the patient to use the finger immediately.

Complication
Division of a digital nerve.

de Quervain's stenosing tenovaginitis

The condition

Stenosing tenovaginitis at the radial styloid is commonly called de Quervain's disease (Fritz de Quervain, Berne surgeon born 1868). It is due to inflammation around the tendons of extensor pollicis brevis and abductor pollicis longus as they pass through the first dorsal extensor compartment over the radial styloid.

Making the diagnosis

The patient
The patient is usually a middle-aged female.

The history
The patient complains of pain just proximal to the anatomical snuff box, which worsens on using the hand.

On examination
There may be a palpable swelling over the tendons. You may be able to elicit tenderness on pressing around the tendons as they pass in their canal.

You may be able to feel crepitus if you feel over the first dorsal compartment and ask the patient to flex and extend their thumb.

Finkelstein's manoeuvre may be used to confirm the diagnosis. This is performed by holding the thumb adducted in the palm while deviating the wrist ulnarwards. This will reproduce the pain. Always compare the two sides.

Treatment

If the patient presents with only a week or two of pain, they should be given some anti-inflammatory medication. Some surgeons prescribe splints but they have not been proven to be effective.

If the patient has had symptoms for more than a few weeks, an injection of local steroid into the canal, around the tendons, is often curative. The injection may fail if the tendons run in two separate compartments. The injection can lead to some depigmentation of the overlying skin. The patient must be warned about this.

Indications for surgery

Persistent symptoms that have not responded to conservative therapy.

Operation: decompression of de Quervain's tenovaginitis

A 2.5 cm (1 inch) longitudinal or transverse incision is made over the tendons. The roof of the canal is divided. Both tendons must be decompressed. If they run in two separate compartments, both must be opened. Care is taken to see and preserve the superficial branches of the radial nerve.

Codes

GA/LA	LA or regional
Blood	0
Antibiotics	0
Time	30 minutes
Drains	0
Plaster	0
Postoperative radiograph	0
Stay	Day case
Follow-up	10 days
Off work	10 days

Postoperative care

Management

- Elevate the hand for the first day postoperatively.
- Encourage the patient to use their thumb immediately.

Complications

- Failure to completely divide the entire sheath may lead to persistent symptoms.
- Division of the superficial radial nerve may leave an anaesthetic area on the dorsum of the thumb and also produce a painful neuroma at the site of the incision.

CHAPTER 39

Dupuytren's contracture

The condition

This is a contracture of the palmar aponeurosis that may progress to a flexion deformity of one or more finger (Baron Guillaume Dupuytren, Paris surgeon born 1777).

Making the diagnosis

The patient

The typical patient is a middle-aged male. He may be of Celtic descent, with pale blue eyes and fair hair. There may be a family history of the disease. The commonly stated association between Dupuytren's and alcoholism is probably spurious. There is a high incidence in epileptics receiving phenytoin therapy and in diabetics.

Dupuytren's contracture can be triggered off by an injury. For example the incidence of Dupuytren's is increased following Colles' fracture. The trauma may be so insignificant that the patient has difficulty recalling the event, such as a minor cut in the hand.

The history

The patient will either complain of a painful nodule in the palm, or of a painless thickening in the palm and the inability to straighten his finger. The latter typically leads to the finger getting caught when putting his hand in his trouser pocket and to the patient poking himself in the eye when washing his face!

On examination

Examine both hands.

Carefully document the location of the fascial bands. They are over the flexor tendons in the palm, but usually go to one or other side of the tendon as they enter the finger.

141

Make a note of the range of movement in the metacarpophalangeal (MCP), proximal interphalangeal (PIP) and distal interphalangeal (DIP) joints for each of the affected fingers. Remember that a full extended joint is at 0° (not at 180°). If the joint does not fully extend, but flexes further then there is a fixed flexion deformity. For example if the MCP joint cannot be straightened beyond 30° but bends to 90° the range of movement is noted as 30–90°.

It is simplest to tabulate the examination as follows:

Left	MCP	PIP	DIP
Index	0–90	0–100	0–80
Middle	0–90	0–100	0–80
Ring	30–90	0–90	0–80
Little	45–90	45–90	30–80

If the patient has had previous surgery, note the position of the scars and examine the sensation in all the fingers to see if the digital nerves are still intact.

Ask the patient to put his hand flat on the table and see if the diseased finger prevents him laying the hand completely flat.

Treatment

Indications for surgery
Surgery is indicated if the contracture prevents the patient laying his palm flat on the table. In severe cases where the tip of the finger is embedded in the palm, amputation of the finger may be the best option.

The patient must be warned that if there is a fixed flexion contracture of the proximal interphalangeal joint due to the Dupuytren's band, that this usually results in abnormality of the joint itself. Therefore after the Dupuytren's bands are excised, the joint may still not fully extend.

The patient must be warned of the risk of digital nerve injury.

Operation: partial (palmar) fasciectomy for Dupuytren's contracture

We make zig-zag skin incisions with the apices at the skin creases of the joints. This is done to avoid the risk of developing a joint contracture that would occur if a straight incision was made across a joint that subsequently contracted.

The abnormal fascial bands are carefully dissected free and removed. The operation effectively is a dissection of the two neuro-vascular bundles. The digital nerve is most at risk as it wraps around the band at the level of the metacarpophalangeal joint. At the end of the procedure the neuro-vascular bundles should remain intact.

If there is a skin contracture, one can either perform Z-plasties to gain extra skin length, or leave the wound open in the palm to close secondarily (McCash open palm technique).

Codes

GA/LA	Regional block or GA
Blood	0
Antibiotics	0
Time	1–2 hours
Drains	Sometimes
Plaster	0
Postoperative radiograph	0
Stay	Day case or one night
Follow-up	10 days
Off work	4 weeks

Operative requirement
High arm tourniquet.

Postoperative care

Management
Elevate the hand for 24 hours.

Check the sensation in the distribution of the digital nerves at risk.

Beware haematoma formation – hand operations are not generally painful postoperatively. If the patient complains of severe pain, remove all the dressings and inspect the wound. If there is a haematoma, remove one or two sutures. This may be enough to allow its evacuation. If this fails, the patient may have to return to theatre to have the haematoma drained.

If a drain is left in the wound it should be removed after 24 hours.

143

If the surgeon is worried about the viability of the skin he should take down the dressings and check that the skin flaps are viable 48 hours postoperatively.

Complications

- Division of a digital nerve.
- Postoperative haematoma.
- Death of a skin flap.
- Residual contracture of the proximal interphalangeal joint.
- Recurrence of the disease is probably inevitable and not truly a complication.

CHAPTER 40

Divided flexor tendons

The condition

Flexor tendons are commonly injured. The injury may be self inflicted and accidental such as when a sharp knife slips. People sometimes punch windows and suffer several lacerations that all need to be explored. Flexor tendon injury may be accompanied by division of a digital nerve and artery.

Flexor tendon injuries are classified according to their location. From the point where the tendons enter their synovial sheath in the palm, until the slips of superficial flexor tendon insert onto the middle phalanx, is called Zone II. This is also known as 'no-man's land' due to the difficulty in getting a good result following tendon repair. Following surgery, adhesions can prevent smooth gliding of the tendon in the canal. This accounts for the difficulty in achieving good results from tendon repair in this Zone II.

Making the diagnosis

The history

Establish the exact mechanism of injury. If the fingers were flexed when cut, as in someone who grasps a knife blade, the tendon ends will be some distance from the original wound when the fingers are extended. The fingers will be held extended on the operating table and retrieval of the tendon ends can be difficult.

Find out what caused the laceration. If caused by glass, you should order a radiograph to see if there is any glass in the wound.

On examination
Look at the patient's hand at rest. Normally fingers rest slightly flexed, but if both flexor tendons to a finger are divided, the injured finger will lie extended.

Examine the function of the superficial flexor and the deep flexor tendon for each finger:

(a) hold all the patient's fingers extended except the one you are examining. Ask the patient to flex the finger that is free. The superficial flexor tendon (FDS) is intact if he can flex the finger at the proximal interphalangeal joint;

(b) to examine the deep flexor (FDP) tendon, hold the proximal interphalangeal joint extended of the finger being examined. Then ask the patient to flex the tip of the finger. Deep flexor function is intact if the patient can flex the distal interphalangeal joint;

(c) a normal variation in the little finger, is the inability to flex the proximal interphalangeal joint of the little finger while the other fingers are held extended. If there is a possibility that the FDS tendon to the little finger has been cut, compare the injured with the uninjured side.

Examine sensation in the fingers and ensure that they have an intact vascularity with good capillary refill at the fingertips.

Radiographs
Radiographs of the hand are essential to exclude a fracture or the presence of a foreign body.

Preoperative management

Common associated injuries
Divided digital nerve or artery.

Preparation for surgery
Clean and then dress the wound with a saline-soaked swab.

If the interval until operation is likely to be more than a few hours, immobilize the hand in a back-slab up to the fingertips, with the wrist and the metacarpophalangeal joints flexed. This may reduce the retraction of the proximal end of the cut tendons.

Give tetanus toxoid if the patient is not fully covered against tetanus.

Treatment

Indications for surgery
Laceration in the hand with a clinical suspicion of a flexor tendon injury.

Contra-indication to surgery
Late presentation, i.e. after more than 48 hours, with a contaminated wound. In these patients, it is better to let the wound heal and perform the exploration as an elective, delayed procedure, 10 days or more after the injury.

Operation: repair of divided flexor tendons in the hand

The laceration is extended in a zig-zag fashion with the apices of the incision at the skin creases of the joints. This avoids the risk of a joint contracture that would occur if a straight incision was used that subsequently contracted.

If the proximal tendon end is not easily found, we often make a separate incision in the palm to allow the tendon to be advanced into the wound. Once retrieved, the tendons are repaired using a meticulous technique to diminish the risk of adhesions within the tendon sheath and a subsequently poor result.

Codes

GA/LA	GA
Blood	0
Antibiotics	Yes
Time	1 hour minimum
Drains	0
Plaster	Below elbow to finger tips
Postoperative radiograph	0
Stay	2 days
Follow-up	1 week
Off work	6 weeks

Operative requirements
High arm tourniquet. The operating microscope should be available in theatre if there is a likelihood of a digital nerve or artery repair.

147

Postoperative care

Management

Mobilization instructions depend on whether dynamic traction with elastic bands, or active and passive mobilization is used.

Some surgeons place an elastic band on the fingertip that goes to a pulley over the wrist. This allows the patient to extend the finger actively and then for the finger to be flexed passively by the elastic band and not the repaired tendons (Kleinert traction). Others instruct the patient on exercises where active extension is permitted, and also gentle active flexion. These regimes of early movement prevent the development of adhesions within the tendon sheath.

If a digital nerve has also been repaired, the finger has to remain flexed for 3 weeks, but passive mobilization can be continued.

The regime for postoperative mobilization should be clearly stated by the surgeon who performed the operation. The patient must understand that his cooperation is vital to obtain a successful result.

The patient must not go home until the dressings have been reduced by the surgeon or hand therapist. Outpatient hand therapy must be arranged prior to the patient's discharge. The patient will need to see the therapist at least weekly for 6 weeks. The surgeon should also see the patient weekly unless he has a hand therapist on whom he can rely to alert him to problems, especially rupture of the tendon repair.

The patient will wear a dorsal splint that prevents MCP joints extending beyond 70° of flexion but allow full extension at the PIP joints. The splint is worn for 6 weeks. Even if only one finger is injured, all the fingers are protected. The patient may not use the hand for heavy lifting for another 2 weeks after the splint is removed.

Complications

- Injury to neuro-vascular bundle in the digit.
- Infection.
- Stiffness.
- Rupture of repaired tendon.

Cut digital nerve

The condition

This is a common hand injury. The digital artery that runs deep to the nerve is often injured as well.

The ulnar side of the little finger, the radial side of the index finger and both sides of the thumb are the most important areas of sensation for hand function.

Remember that a digital nerve contains 6000 nerve fibres and is easily seen with the naked eye.

Making the diagnosis

The patient

The age of the patient may influence the decision to operate or not. Children can regain normal sensation after repair of a nerve and so injured nerves are almost always repaired. The recovery is not very good beyond middle age and surgery may not be justified. Find out whether the patient is left or right-handed. Ask an adult about their occupation and hobbies.

The history

If there was profuse bleeding from a cut on the side of the finger it is likely that the digital artery is cut. If the artery has been cut, it is practically inevitable that the nerve is divided since the nerve lies superficial to the artery.

Find out exactly how the finger was injured and with what. A laceration from a sharp knife will divide a nerve cleanly without loss of any nerve substance. Injury from circular saw may remove a segment of nerve. If more than a few millimetres of nerve have been lost, end to end repair may not be possible.

On examination

Examine sensation in the normal areas and compare this to sensation in the area supplied by the potentially injured nerve. Just examine for light touch and do not repeatedly stick sharp needles into the fingers to test pain sensation. Remember that it is possible to have some slight sensation even after complete division of a nerve. The most reliable sign of complete division of the nerve, is loss of sweating in the area supplied by the nerve. Compare the dryness of the skin of the fingers.

Always test and document flexor tendon function.

Radiographs

If the laceration was caused by glass, order a radiograph to see if there is any radio-opaque glass in the wound. Remember certain types of glass do not show up on radiographs.

Preoperative management

Common associated injuries

Flexor tendon injury.

Preparation for surgery

Once you have performed a careful and thorough examination, clean the wound and cover it with a dressing soaked in an antiseptic such as aqueous Betadine. Do not allow lots of different people to repeatedly remove the dressing to look at the wound.

You must warn the patient that a repaired nerve may take 3 years to reach the end point of recovery. The patient must realize that sensation after a nerve repair is never normal.

Treatment

Indications for surgery

A divided digital nerve that is suitable for repair. It is not feasible to repair a nerve that is divided beyond the level of the distal interphalangeal joint.

If the nerves to the thumb, or the radial side of index finger or the ulnar side of the little finger are divided they should be repaired if at all possible. This is to provide protective sensation to the vulnerable areas of the digits.

Operation: digital nerve repair

The wound is extended in a zig-zag fashion. The apices of the incision are at the skin creases of the joints. This avoids the risk of a joint contracture that would occur if a straight incision was used that subsequently contracted.

The nerve is repaired using microsurgical sutures. Some surgeons use a fibrin glue to minimize the number of sutures used.

Codes

GA/LA	GA or regional block
Blood	0
Antibiotics	Yes
Time	1 hour
Drains	0
Plaster	Below elbow dorsal slab to the finger tips
Postoperative radiograph	0
Stay	1 night
Follow-up	10 days
Off work	3 weeks minimum

Operative requirements

- Microsurgical instruments.
- Operating microscope or magnifying loupes.
- Fibrin glue.

Postoperative care

Management

- Elevate the hand overnight.
- The plaster slab is kept on for 3 weeks.

Complications

- Failure of nerve recovery.
- Many patients experience a period of hypersensitivity that lasts for up to a year.
- Adults never regain normal sensation, only good 'abnormal' sensation.

Divided extensor tendon

The condition

This is a common injury. Usually the tendon is divided by a sharp object such as a knife or piece of glass.

Extensor tendons heal with much less problem than flexor tendons. Indeed, if a finger is held extended with a splint, the tendon can heal without surgery. However, wounds need to be cleaned and it is often a simple matter to repair the tendon.

Making the diagnosis

The patient
Ask the patient about his occupation and his hobbies. Which is the patient's dominant hand?

The history
Document how and when the injury occurred. If the laceration is over the metacarpophalangeal joint as a result of the patient punching an opponent in the mouth, the joint itself may be contaminated.

On examination
Test active extension of the MCP joints separate from the PIP and DIP joints. Remember that the intrinsic muscles extend the PIP and DIP joints. When an extensor tendon is divided proximal to the MCP joint, the patient will still be able to extend the PIP and DIP joints once you hold the MCP joint extended. Also remember that there are independent extensors to the index and the little fingers.

Radiographs

Radiographs of the hand are essential to exclude a fracture and to look for a foreign body in the wound. A piece of the opponent's tooth will easily be seen on the radiograph!

Preoperative management

Preparation for surgery

Once you have performed a careful and thorough examination, clean the wound and cover it with a dressing soaked in an antiseptic such as aqueous Betadine. Do not allow lots of different people to repeatedly remove the dressing to look at the wound.

Give the patient tetanus toxoid if they are not fully covered against tetanus.

Treatment

Indications for surgery

A wound on the hand with a possible extensor tendon injury.

Operation: repair of divided extensor tendon

The wound is extended to obtain a clear view. If the tendon is divided, it is repaired.

If the wound is near the MCP joint, the joint must be assumed to be contaminated. The joint must explored and washed out thoroughly.

Codes

GA/LA	GA or regional block
Blood	0
Antibiotics	Yes
Time	1 hour
Drains	0
Plaster	Volar slab
Postoperative radiograph	0
Stay	1 night post operation
Follow-up	10 days
Off work	2–6 weeks

Operative requirement
High arm tourniquet.

Postoperative care

Management
If an extensor tendon is repaired proximal to the MCP joints, the plaster slab only needs to extend up to the PIP joints. If the repair is on the dorsum of the finger itself, only the finger is kept extended. The plaster is kept on for 3 or 4 weeks.

Complications
Wound infection.

43 Infection in the hand

The condition

Infection in the hand that results in a collection of pus can cause diagnostic and therapeutic problems. Pus may be localized in the midpalmar and thenar spaces in the hand, or may track along the tendon sheaths from a finger into the palm and wrist.

Making the diagnosis

The history

The patient may have had a minor puncture wound that initially went unnoticed. He may be in an occupation that has a high risk of infection.

The patient will complain of increasing pain in the hand that may become excruciating. The patient may be systemically unwell.

Ask about a family history of diabetes, as infection may be the first presentation of the disease.

On examination

The patient's temperature must be measured.

If the infection is in a deep space in the hand, the hand will be swollen, red and exquisitely tender. Due to the unforgiving nature of the palmar fascia, the swelling may be maximal on the dorsum of the hand.

With a tendon sheath infection, the affected finger will be red, swollen and held flexed. Any movement of the finger, either actively or passively, is exceedingly painful. You must examine the palm and the wrist for tenderness. This is because the infection can track down the tendon sheath. In the thumb and the little finger, the sheath is continuous with the bursae in the wrist. The sheaths of the middle three fingers open into the palm.

Radiographs
Order radiographs of the hand and fingers to exclude a foreign body or underlying osteomyelitis.

Preoperative management

Investigations
These must include a full blood count and ESR. If the patient's pyrexia is greater than 38°C, take blood cultures.

If you are at all suspicious of the infection being the first presentation of diabetes, measure the blood glucose.

Preparation for surgery
Rest the hand in a back-slab and elevate.

Treatment

Indications for surgery
- A localized collection of pus that is not draining spontaneously.
- Tendon sheath infection.

Operation: incision and drainage of hand infection

For a palmar space infection, the incision is made directly over the abscess.

For a tendon sheath infection, a lateral incision is made in the fingertip and a transverse one in the palm, so that the tendon sheath can be irrigated.

Codes

GA/LA	GA
Blood	0
Antibiotics	Start after a specimen of pus has been obtained
Time	30 minutes
Drains	0
Plaster	Below-elbow volar slab up to fingertips
Postoperative radiograph	0
Stay	3–4 days

| Follow-up | 2 days |
| Off work | 2 weeks |

Operative requirements

Have a tourniquet on the upper arm, but try to avoid its use. If a tourniquet is used, exsanguinate the limb by elevation only. Send a specimen of pus for immediate Gram stain and culture. Once the specimen has been taken, start intravenous flucloxacillin ± Fucidin until the sensitivities are available. If the entry wound was due to a punch injury from an opponent's teeth, add metronidazole.

Postoperative care

Management

Immobilize the whole hand in a volar slab with the metacarpophalangeal joints at 70°, and the proximal interphalangeal and distal interphalangeal joints extended, until the infection has completely resolved.

Elevate the upper limb.

Obtain microbiology results as soon as possible and if necessary, change the antibiotic regime.

Complications

Inadequate drainage and debridement resulting in re-accumulation of pus.

CHAPTER

44

Fractured metacarpal

The condition

The metacarpal may fracture at the neck, through the shaft or at the base.

Making the diagnosis

The history

Punching a solid object, falling onto a clenched fist or a direct blow to the hand are the usual causes of a metacarpal fracture. The patient complains of pain and swelling around the fracture.

It is important to know the dominant hand and the occupation of the patient. The patient's age is also a consideration, as one may accept displacement in an 80-year-old that you would not in a 20-year-old.

On examination

It is vital that you look for a rotational deformity. This is best done by asking the patient to slowly flex the fingers. If pain inhibits active flexion by the patient, you should passively and gently flex all the fingers together. Normally all the fingers will point toward the scaphoid, without over or under-lapping. Always compare the injured hand with the normal hand.

Examine the distal circulation of the injured finger (capillary refill) and look for evidence of a nerve injury.

Radiographs

The whole hand.

158

Preoperative management

Preparation for surgery

Immobilize the hand in a below-elbow volar slab, with the metacarpophalangeal joints at 70° and the fingers straight.

Treatment

The majority of metacarpal fractures are treated as outpatients. The aim of treatment is to maintain hand function rather than obtain perfect radiographs. Undisplaced fractures and those with acceptable angulation on the lateral view do not require anything more than immobilization for 2–3 weeks. The amount of acceptable angulation (on the lateral view) increases from 15° for the index metacarpal to 30° for the fifth metacarpal. Give the patient a Bedford splint to wear. This is a removable double tube that functions as neighbour strapping.

Simple transverse or oblique fractures may need closed manipulation and the insertion of percutaneous K-wires.

More comminuted fractures may need open reduction and internal fixation either with screws alone or with a plate and screws.

Indications for surgery

A rotational deformity is an absolute indication for surgery. If there is considerable shortening of the metacarpal, especially of the index finger, surgery is often necessary.

Operation: metacarpal fracture
1. Closed reduction and K-wiring
2. Open reduction and internal fixation

1. Under image intensification, the fracture is reduced and then held with one or two K-wires passed percutaneously. It is often simplest to pass the wires transversely through the fractured metacarpal into the adjacent metacarpal. This holds the fractured metacarpal out to length and in the correct rotation. The wires are left with their ends exposed to allow them to be removed on follow up in the clinic.

2. The fracture is reduced through an incision on the dorsum of the hand. It is then held with either screws alone, or screws and a plate.

159

Codes

GA/LA	GA or regional block
Blood	0
Antibiotics	Yes
Time	1 hour
Drains	0
Plaster	Yes
Postoperative radiograph	AP and lateral hand
Stay	One night or day case
Follow-up	2 weeks
Off work	6 weeks

Operative requirements
- Mini-fragment AO set and/or K-wire set.
- Tourniquet.
- Image intensifier and radiographer.

Postoperative care

Management
Elevate the hand for 24 hours.

The duration of plaster immobilization depends on the rigidity of the fixation and must be specified by the surgeon. Ideally the fixation should be rigid enough to start immediate, gentle, active mobilization.

Complications
- Infection.
- Loss of position.
- Reduced range of movement of the finger due to adhesion of the extensor tendons to the plate.

45 Rupture of the ulnar collateral ligament of the thumb (gamekeeper's thumb)

The condition

Injury to the ulnar collateral ligament of the metacarpophalangeal joint of the thumb may be a sprain or a complete rupture. Originally described as an overuse laxity in gamekeepers, the term 'gamekeeper's thumb' is nowadays used to describe an acute injury.

Making the diagnosis

The history

This injury results from sudden dorsiflexion and abduction of the thumb. It is common after a fall on a dry ski slope, where the thumb gets caught in a hole in the mat, or during a fall while snow skiing when the thumb is wrenched by the strap of the ski pole. It is sometimes called ski-pole thumb.

The patient complains of pain around the ulnar side of the metacarpophalangeal joint of the thumb. They may also have noticed a weakness in pinch grip. This is due to the lack of stability of the metacarpophalangeal joint of the thumb.

On examination

There is tenderness around the ulnar side of the metacarpophalangeal joint. There may be some swelling or a bruise.

Hold the metacarpophalangeal joint extended and then radially deviate the proximal phalanx. If the ulnar collateral ligament is intact you will reach a definite end point after a little bit of give. If the ligament is not intact you are able to open the joint abnormally.

Make sure that you examine the other thumb to establish the normal laxity of the ligament. Always document the range of flexion of the metacarpophalangeal joint for that patient for both the injured and the normal thumb.

The range of flexion at the metacarpophalangeal joint varies tremendously. Some people can only flex to 30° but others can flex to 90°. People with stiff metacarpophalangeal joints are more likely to suffer injury to the thumb.

Radiographs

Radiographs of the thumb may show a bone fragment avulsed from the ulnar corner of the proximal phalanx.

If the diagnosis is in doubt, stress films can be taken comparing the two thumbs.

It is possible to assess the integrity of the ligament with an ultrasound.

Treatment

If the ligament is sprained, or the fracture of the base of the proximal phalanx is undisplaced, immobilize the thumb in a plaster cast for 4 weeks.

Indications for surgery

Complete rupture of the ulnar collateral ligament.

Avulsion of the bony insertion of the ligament with displacement of the bony fragment.

Operation: open repair of the ulnar collateral ligament of the thumb

The joint is exposed through a 3 cm dorso-medial incision over the joint.

If the bone fragment is big enough, it may be held with a mini-fragment screw. If it is small, a suture is passed from the ligament through the proximal phalanx. The suture is brought out through the skin and tied over a button on the radial side of the thumb. The suture is pulled out after four weeks.

If the ligament is ruptured in its mid-substance, the two ends are sutured together. If the rupture is old, it may be necessary to use a tendon graft from palmaris longus to reconstruct the ligament.

Following repair, the joint may be immobilized by a K-wire.

Codes

GA/LA	GA or regional block
Blood	0
Antibiotics	Optional
Time	45 minutes
Drains	0
Plaster	Thumb spica
Postoperative radiograph	AP and lateral MCP joint only if bone fixed
Stay	One night
Follow-up	10 days
Off work	6 weeks

Operative requirements
- Mini-fragment AO set or small K-wire set.
- Tourniquet.
- Small air-powered drill.

Postoperative care

Management
- Elevate the hand while an inpatient.
- The plaster is kept on for 4 weeks.

Complications
- Division of dorsal branch of the radial nerve.
- Stiff metacarpophalangeal joint.

46 Bennett's fracture-dislocation of the thumb

The condition

This is a fracture of the base of the first metacarpal that is intra-articular. The volar (palmar) fracture fragment stays in place, but the shaft subluxates or dislocates dorsally off the trapezium (E. H. Bennett born 1837, Dublin surgeon).

Making the diagnosis

The history
The injury occurs following violent extension of the thumb. The injury may occur following a fall or during a contact sport such as rugby. The patient has pain just distal to the anatomical snuff box.

On examination
There is usually tenderness around the base of the metacarpal. You may feel instability and crepitus on extending the thumb.

Radiographs
Request AP and lateral radiographs of the metacarpophalangeal joint of the thumb. The palmar corner of the base of metacarpal remains in place on the trapezium. If the fracture is displaced, the rest of the metacarpal is dislocated dorsally from the trapezium.

Treatment

If the fracture is undisplaced, it is not a Bennett's fracture-dislocation and the thumb can be immobilized in a scaphoid-type plaster cast. If there is a dislocation, it must be reduced and then held.

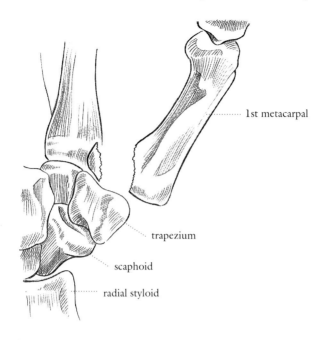

1st metacarpal

trapezium

scaphoid

radial styloid

Indications for surgery

As this is an intra-articular fracture, accurate reduction is required. This may be possible by closed manipulation and percutaneous K-wiring. If this is unsuccessful, an open reduction is performed and the fracture position held with K-wires.

Operation: Bennett's fracture-dislocation of the thumb
1. Manipulation under anaesthesia ± K-wiring
2. Open reduction and K-wiring

1. Under screening with the image intensifier, it may be possible to reduce the fracture by closed manipulation and hold the position with a padded cast. The thumb is immobilized in extension with pressure on the base of the first metacarpal. Alternatively, the position can be held with K-wires inserted percutaneously.

2. If closed reduction is not successful, a dorsal incision is made over the base of the metacarpal. The fracture is reduced and held with K-wires.

Codes

GA/LA	GA or regional block
Blood	0
Antibiotics	Yes, if open reduction
Time	1 hour
Drains	0
Plaster	Scaphoid cast
Postoperative radiograph	AP and lateral thumb
Stay	One night
Follow-up	1 week, X-ray on arrival
Off work	6 weeks

Operative requirements

- Image intensifier and radiographer.
- K-wire set and powered driver.

Postoperative care

Management

- The arm should be elevated for the first 24 hours.
- K-wires are removed after 5 weeks, in the clinic.

Complication

Failure to achieve anatomical reduction.

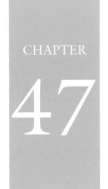

CHAPTER

47

Fracture of the phalanx

The condition

A phalanx may fracture through one or both condyles involving the PIP or DIP joint, through the shaft or at the base. Fractures may be simple or comminuted.

Making the diagnosis

The history

A punch, falling onto a clenched fist or a direct blow are the usual causes of a phalangeal fracture. The patient will complain of pain and swelling around the fracture.

It is important to know the dominant hand and the occupation of the patient. The age is also a consideration, as one may accept displacement in an 80-year-old that you would not accept in a 20-year-old.

On examination

Look at the finger when in extension. Any angular deformity should be obvious.

A rotational deformity is harder to detect. Ask the patient to slowly flex the fingers. If pain inhibits active flexion by the patient, you should passively and gently flex the fingers. If there is no rotational deformity, all the fingers will point towards the scaphoid, without over- or under-lapping. If there is abnormal rotation that is not corrected, a rotational malunion will result. This can lead to a severe functional problem. Always compare the injured hand with the normal hand.

Radiographs

AP and lateral views of the fingers.

Preoperative management

Preparation for surgery
Immobilize the hand in a below elbow volar slab, with the meta-carpophalangeal joints at 70° and the fingers straight.

Treatment

The aim of treatment is to obtain the best functional result possible. We treat the patient rather than the patient's radiographs. Open operation on a finger is more likely to result in postoperative stiffness than closed methods of treatment. The risk of stiffness is increased if the finger is immobilized for several weeks following surgery.

The decision to operate rather than to treat conservatively depends on balancing the risks of surgery against the result of conservative treatment and early mobilization.

Indications for surgery
An intra-articular fracture with more than a millimetre of displacement requires reduction and fixation.

A fractured shaft with a rotational or angular deformity should have the deformity corrected and the fracture stabilized.

There are a variety of techniques for stabilizing small bone fractures. These include a mini-external fixator, percutaneous K-wires, mini-fragment screws alone or (rarely) mini-fragment plates and screws.

Operation: phalangeal fracture
1. Closed reduction and percutaneous K-wiring
2. Open reduction and internal fixation
3. Closed reduction and external fixation

1. The finger is manipulated and the fracture reduced. One or two fine K-wires are inserted to hold the fracture fragments in place. The position of the fracture and wires is checked with the image intensifier. The wires are usually left just under or just through the skin.
2. The exact site of the incision depends on the fracture. Generally the incision is lateral or dorsal. The fracture is reduced under direct vision and then held either with one or two screws alone, or with a plate and screws.

3. If the fracture is comminuted, it may not be possible to fix the fracture directly. A mini-external fixator can be placed with both pins in the proximal phalanx, or with one pin in the proximal phalanx and one pin in the middle phalanx for an intra-articular fracture. The position of the fracture is checked with the image intensifier.

Codes

GA/LA	GA or regional block
Blood	0
Antibiotics	Yes
Time	1 hour
Drains	0
Plaster	Possibly
Postoperative radiograph	Yes
Stay	Day case or 1 night post operation
Follow-up	10 days
Off work	2–6 weeks, depending on the fixation and the patient's occupation

Operative requirements

- AO mini-fragment set, K-wire set and small powered drill.
- Tourniquet.
- Image intensifier.

Postoperative care

Management
Elevate the hand following surgery.

If the fixation is strong enough, the surgeon may want the patient to start gently moving the finger immediately. If the fixation is not very strong, the finger may need to be protected in a plaster cast for a few weeks.

Percutaneous wires and external fixators are taken off in the outpatient clinic after 4 weeks.

Complications
- Infection.
- Stiffness of the finger.
- Loss of position.

CHAPTER 48

Rheumatoid arthritis affecting the hand

The condition

The hands are commonly involved in rheumatoid arthritis. The exact pattern of involvement is variable. Usually the changes are bilateral and symmetrical.

Synovitis over the dorsum of the hand is common. This itself can be painful. The synovitis may secondarily lead to destruction of extensor tendons. Bony prominences, such as a large ulnar head, can also lead to extensor tendon rupture. The extensor tendons to the little and ring fingers usually rupture first. The destruction may continue and the thumb extensor and the extensors to the middle and index fingers may also rupture.

There are other causes of lack of active finger extension. These include 'dislocation' of the extensor mechanism off the metacarpal head into the valley in between the metacarpal heads, or a posterior interosseous nerve palsy.

Rheumatoid arthritis commonly affects the metacarpophalangeal joints. The fingers may develop ulnar drift due to soft tissue disease only. The metacarpophalangeal joints themselves may become destroyed and dislocate.

Making the diagnosis

The patient
The patient usually has problems throughout the upper limbs. The hands should not be considered in isolation from the shoulders and elbows.

The history
In your assessment you should distinguish between the complaint of pain and the complaint of loss of function. Always enquire as to how

the patient manages everyday activities, such as holding a cup of tea, doing up buttons and zips, etc.

If the patient cannot extend a finger actively, find out if this occurred as an acute event or if this came on gradually. Also ask if there was preceding swelling over the dorsum of the hand and wrist suggestive of synovitis.

If the patient has marked ulna drift of the fingers, ask what bothers them most. It may be the appearance, or the pain around the metacarpophalangeal joints or poor grip, or all three.

On examination

Examine the passive movements of the wrist and fingers. If there is ulnar drift of the fingers, see if you can bring the fingers back into a normal position. Try to feel the metacarpophalangeal joints to see if they are dislocated.

If the patient cannot extend a finger try to distinguish between the causes given above. A prominent ulna styloid should be noted. See if the extensor mechanism is located over the metacarpal head. If it is not, put the finger into extension and then ask the patient to hold their finger extended.

Radiographs

AP and lateral views of the hand.

Preoperative management

Investigations

As with all patients with rheumatoid arthritis undergoing surgery, check that they have a good range of neck movement and can open their mouth wide. Ensure that there is a recent set of radiographs of the cervical spine.

Treatment – ruptured extensor tendon(s)

Indications for surgery

End to end repair is not possible if an extensor tendon is ruptured due to rheumatoid arthritis. A tendon transfer combined with a synovectomy of the dorsum of the wrist usually gives excellent results. The synovectomy is performed to try to prevent further tendon ruptures. If the ulnar head is prominent then it should be excised.

Operation: tendon transfer for ruptured extensor tendons

We make an incision on the dorsum of the wrist. The abnormal synovium around the extensors tendons is excised. If prominent, the ulnar head is excised. We place part or all of the extensor retinaculum under the extensor tendons to try to prevent further ruptures.

If only a single extensor is ruptured, we transfer the extensor indicis to provide power. Active index finger extension remains using extensor communis. (Remember that extensor indicis is the more ulnar of the two extensor tendons to the index finger.) We use a small incision over the index metacarpal head and one over the little finger metacarpal head in addition to the main incision.

We use a variety of transfers if more than one tendon is ruptured.

Codes

GA/LA	GA or regional block
Blood	0
Antibiotics	0
Time	1 hour
Drains	Yes
Plaster	Palmar slab up to the proximal interphalangeal joints for 4 weeks post operation
Postoperative radiograph	0
Stay	1 night post operation
Follow-up	10 days
Off work	2 weeks minimum, depending on job

Operative requirements

- Small saw.
- High arm tourniquet.

Postoperative care

Management

The palmar slab extends only up to the proximal interphalangeal joints to allow the patient to extend the PIP and DIP joints using their intrinsic muscles. The slab is worn for 4 weeks. Active mobilization is then supervised by the physiotherapist.

Complications

- Tendon transfer too tight so some flexion is lost.
- Tendon transfer is too loose so that an extensor lag persists.

Treatment – ulnar drift of the fingers

Indications for surgery

Severe ulnar drift of the fingers with well-preserved metacarpophalangeal joints on the radiographs.

Operation: soft tissue correction of ulnar drift of the fingers (intrinsic transfer)

We make a transverse incision across the dorsum of the metacarpophalangeal joints. The tendon of the ulnar intrinsic to the index, middle and ring fingers, and the abductor digiti minimi are divided. The ulnar intrinsic to the index is transferred to the radial side of the middle finger and so on for the middle, ring and little fingers. The transfer reduces the ulnar pull on each finger and increases the pull in the radial direction. We may also rebalance the extensor mechanism over the metacarpal head.

Codes

GA/LA	GA
Blood	0
Antibiotics	0
Time	1 hour
Drains	Yes
Plaster	Palmar slab to keep the fingers in their corrected position
Postoperative radiograph	0
Stay	2–3 days
Follow-up	10 days
Off work	2 weeks minimum

Operative requirement

High arm tourniquet.

Postoperative care

Management

The patient should be fitted with two splints within a few days of surgery. The patient must not go home until the splints are fitted and are checked by the surgeon. A dynamic extension splint that allows MCP joint flexion, but pulls the fingers back into a slightly over-corrected position, is worn during the day. A fixed splint which holds the fingers extended in a slightly over corrected position is worn at night. The splints are worn for 6 weeks following surgery.

Complication

Recurrence of the ulnar drift.

Treatment – MCP joint dislocation and ulnar drift of the fingers

Indications for surgery

If the patient has severe ulnar drift of the fingers and destroyed MCP joints on the radiographs, MCP joint replacement is a reliable procedure.

Operation: replacement of the metacarpophalangeal joints

We make a transverse incision over dorsum of the metacarpophalangeal joints. The head of the metacarpal is removed and the base of the proximal phalanx opened. We insert a plastic hinge to replace the joint. We usually rebalance the fingers and we may include an intrinsic transfer (see above).

Codes

GA/LA	GA
Blood	0
Antibiotics	Yes
Time	1 hour
Drains	Yes
Plaster	Palmar slab to keep the fingers in their corrected position
Postoperative radiograph	0
Stay	2–3 days

Follow-up   10 days
Off work   2 weeks minimum

Operative requirements
- High arm tourniquet.
- Small power saw.
- Silastic MCP joints.

Postoperative care

Management
The patient should be fitted with two splints within a few days of surgery. A dynamic extension splint that allows MCP joint flexion, but pulls the fingers back into a slightly over-corrected position is worn during the day. A fixed splint that holds the fingers extended in a slightly over corrected position is worn at night. The splints are worn for 6 weeks following surgery.

Complications
- Wound infection.
- Dislocation of the artificial joint.
- Fragmentation or loosening of the prosthesis.

Arthritis around the trapezium

The condition

This is often called CMC (carpometacarpal) arthritis of the thumb. The arthritis may involve both the joint between the scaphoid and the trapezium and the joint between the trapezium and the first metacarpal. This is called pan-trapezial arthritis. Alternatively only the joint between the trapezium and the first metacarpal may be affected. The arthritis is commonly bilateral.

Making the diagnosis

The patient
The patient is usually middle-aged. Arthritis at the base of the thumb is more common in women than men.

The history
The patient complains of pain at the base of her thumb. The pain is made worse on use of the thumb, especially when gripping or squeezing. The patient may complain of a lump at the base of the thumb. The lump is caused by a combination of an osteophyte and subluxation of the metacarpal.

Always ask if the patient has symptoms suggesting carpal tunnel syndrome. Both conditions are common in this age group and can occur together.

On examination
Gently palpate the base of the thumb to find out exactly where the patient has pain. It is important to distinguish pain at the CMC joint from pain of de Quervain's tenosynovitis (which is more proximal). Circumduct the thumb to see if this reproduces the pain and at the same time note any crepitus.

Radiographs
Ask for views of the thumb to show the trapezium.

Treatment – pantrapezial arthritis

All possible modes of conservative treatment should be tried before resorting to surgery. These include non-steroidal anti-inflammatory medication, injection of local steroid into the CMC joint and splints.

Indications for surgery
If the patient complains of persistent pain and conservative treatment has failed, surgery should be considered.

Operation: excision of the trapezium and or tendon interposition arthroplasty

The incision is on the dorsum of the hand over the trapezium. If a tendon interposition arthroplasty is performed, additional small incisions are made on the palmar aspect of the wrist. This is so that the flexor carpi radialis tendon can be partially divided and brought into the main wound. The trapezium is removed. In younger patients, the space left after the trapezium has been removed is filled with rolled up tendon.

Codes

GA/LA	GA
Blood	0
Antibiotics	Yes
Time	1 hour
Drains	0
Plaster	Thumb spica
Postoperative radiograph	0
Stay	1 night post operation
Follow-up	10 days
Off work	4 weeks

Operative requirement
Tourniquet.

Postoperative care

Management
The thumb is immobilized in a cast for 3 weeks.

Complications
- Wound infection.
- The silastic replacement can dislocate.
- The silastic replacement can fragment and cause synovitis. This may require removal of the prosthesis.

Treatment – arthritis of the first metacarpophalangeal joint

If the degenerative change is confined to the joint between the trapezium and the metacarpal, this joint can be fused. This gives very little restriction of thumb mobility.

Indications for surgery
Surgery should be considered if the patient complains of persistent pain and conservative treatment has failed.

Operation: arthrodesis of the first carpo-metacarpophalangeal joint

We make an incision over the dorsum of the thumb. The surfaces of the trapezium and the metacarpal are denuded of articular cartilage. The two bones are held together using a screw or a K-wire.

Codes

GA/LA	GA
Blood	0
Antibiotics	Yes
Time	1 hour
Drains	0
Plaster	Thumb spica
Postoperative radiograph	AP and lateral of the thumb
Stay	1 night post operation
Follow-up	10 days
Off work	4 weeks

Operative requirements

- Tourniquet.
- Small cannulated screw set or K-wire set.

Postoperative care

Management

The thumb is immobilized for 4 weeks. If a K-wire has been used, it is removed after 4 weeks.

Complications

- Infection.
- Failure of fusion.
- Unsatisfactory position of thumb fusion.

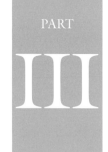

PART

III

Spinal Column

Fracture of a cervical vertebra

The condition

Fractures of the cervical vertebrae include:

1. Flexion or extension injuries where the only bony abnormality is a small piece of bone avulsed from the upper or lower anterior borders of the vertebral body.

2. A major fracture that includes the posterior elements and is unstable.

3. A fracture with retropulsion of fragments into the bony canal resulting in injury to the spinal cord.

4. A fracture of the odontoid peg that is unstable.

One or both facet joints at a single level may dislocate without a fracture.

Making the diagnosis

The patient

A patient who is conscious with a significant neck injury, will have severe pain in the neck and spasm of the paracervical muscles. While conscious the patient is relatively safe from suffering further injury, due to this protective spasm. (The protective spasm is lost should the patient become unconscious or be given a general anaesthetic.)

An unconscious patient who has had significant trauma of any type, especially a blow to the head, must be presumed to have an unstable cervical spine injury until proved otherwise. If there is cervical spine injury, the unconscious patient lacks protective spasm. The spinal cord can be injured if the neck is not kept immobilized.

The history

Cervical fractures are common after direct trauma, such as diving into a shallow pool. They can also occur with indirect trauma such as the rapid flexion and extension when the patient is in a car that collides head-on with another car.

On examination

On a conscious cooperative patient, gently examine the active range of the movements of the neck – flexion/extension, lateral flexion and rotation – and express them as a percentage of those of a normal person.

In a conscious or unconscious patient perform a complete neurological examination of the upper and lower limbs, i.e. sensation, motor power, reflexes, and plantar responses. Check the patient's rectal tone and perianal sensation.

Radiographs

The minimum view that is acceptable is a lateral of the whole cervical spine. The C7/T1 junction *must* be seen. You may have to pull down on the patient's arms to draw down the shoulders while the radiograph is taken, or ask for a swimmer's view (with the arm nearest the X-ray tube extended above the patient's head). If this does not show the C7/T1 junction, you need to obtain either lateral tomograms or a CT scan.

If flexion and extension views are required to exclude instability, they should only be performed on an awake cooperative patient. A doctor should supervise the examination, which must be discontinued if the patient has any abnormal symptoms, such as tingling in the upper or lower limbs.

If a facet dislocation or unstable fracture is suspected, oblique views are required followed by either lateral tomograms or a CT scan or both.

Preoperative management

Prior to definitive management, the neck must be immobilized with a well-fitting stiff collar.

Treatment

If the fracture is stable, immobilization in a well-fitting stiff collar is often adequate.

If there is a fracture that is unstable but is in an acceptable position, the spine must be immobilized. This can be achieved by either skull traction, a halo-vest or a Minerva jacket.

If there is significant displacement of a fracture or an unstable injury, this must be reduced either by traction, by manipulation under anaesthesia or by open operation. Once reduced, the position must be maintained until healing has occurred.

Indications for skeletal traction
An unstable neck fracture or a facet dislocation in an adult.

Contra-indications to skeletal traction
Children and the very elderly, whose skulls are too soft.

Operation: application of skeletal skull traction

A simple and safe means of applying traction is with 'cone callipers'. The pins are inserted 2.5 cm (1 inch) above the top of the ear.

Alternatively, a halo can be applied. This has the advantage of being able to connect the halo to a vest later on. A halo has four pins that go into the skull.

The site for each pin is infiltrated with local anaesthetic down to and including the periosteum. You do not need to shave the hair. The pins are designed with a shoulder to prevent penetration of the inner table of the skull. They are usually supplied with a torque screwdriver that stops you inserting the pins with too much force.

Codes

GA/LA	LA
Blood	0
Antibiotics	0
Time	30 minutes
Drains	0
Plaster	0
Postoperative radiograph	See below

Operative requirements
- Skull traction can be applied in the casualty department.
- Local anaesthetic (1% lignocaine with adrenaline).
- Two doctors.
- Complete set of traction equipment.
- Traction bed.

Postoperative care

Management

For cervical fractures apply 2.25 kg (5 lb) of traction.

For a cervical facet dislocation, start with 2.25 kg (5 lb) traction and obtain a radiograph as soon as the patient is in traction. If still dislocated, increase the weight immediately by 0.5–1 kg (1–2 lb) and obtain a repeat radiograph within the hour. Repeat this increase in weight, followed by a repeat radiograph, until the dislocation is reduced. Once the dislocation is reduced, decrease the traction to 2.25 kg (5 lb).

Complications

The inner table of the skull may be perforated by applying excessive torque to the pins, putting pins into a pathologically porotic skull or misplacing the pins.

Subsequent pin tract infection can lead to meningitis.

CHAPTER 51

Acute low back pain and sciatica

The condition

The cause of acute low back pain is often obscure. However, it can be due to a muscle sprain, or local facet joint disease.

Prolapse of an intervertebral disc usually occurs as an acute event accompanied by the onset of severe sciatica (pain down the back of the leg in the distribution of the sciatic nerve). The disc prolapse is usually lateral but may be central. This rare central disc protrusion does not necessarily produce sciatica but may press on the nerves supplying the sacral plexus and cause irreversible damage to bowel and bladder function.

The investigation of a patient with severe back pain without sciatica must exclude inflammatory causes such as ankylosing spondylitis, external pressure on the vertebrae such as an aortic aneurysm, and bony disease that may be benign or malignant, primary or secondary.

Making the diagnosis

The patient

Acute disc prolapse typically occurs in adults between 20 and 40 years. Elderly patients do not usually suffer disc prolapse as discs become desiccated with ageing. Back pain without sciatica can occur at any age.

The history

Find out if the patient has had episodes of pure back pain prior to suffering sciatica. The back pain may represent weakening of the annular ligament that then ruptures, giving rise to the disc prolapse and sciatica.

Is this the first episode of sciatica? If the patient has suffered sciatica before, how long did the severe pain last? Is this episode as severe as previous episodes?

If the patient has back pain *and* leg pain, ask what percentage of the pain is from the back and what percentage is from the leg.

Establish whether the sciatica radiates down to, or below, the knee. If the pain goes to the foot, does it go to the big toe (L5 dermatome) or to the little toe (S1 dermatome).

What makes the leg pain worse? Of note is laughing, coughing, sneezing, or straining at stool. All of these are associated with an increase in intradural pressure.

Is there any bladder or bowel dysfunction?

What pain killers does the patient take and how often?

Does the pain wake the patient or prevent him from sleeping?

On examination

The examination must include a general examination to exclude a primary malignant disease.

Perform a complete neurological examination of the lower limbs.

Look for signs of nerve root irritation, i.e. a limited straight-leg raise that produces sciatica that increases with dorsiflexion of the ankle, or internal rotation of the hip or pressure on the popliteal nerve. A crossed-leg sign (sciatica when the contralateral straight-leg raise is performed) is also a reliable indicator of a disc protrusion.

Wasting of the extensor digitorum brevis is a reliable sign of a L5 root lesion. Loss of ankle reflex indicates an S1 lesion.

Do not omit a rectal examination. Lack of perianal sensation and poor rectal tone may indicate a central disc protrusion. This is rare, but is a surgical emergency and must be decompressed as soon as possible to preserve bladder and bowel function.

Radiographs

AP and lateral views of the lumbo-sacral spine (these are invariably normal in a patient with a disc protrusion).

An MR scan is the best investigation for a patient with sciatica. Some patients are not suitable for undergoing an MR scan. The patient cannot have an MR scan if they have metal implants (orthopaedic fixation devices or a pacemaker for example), or they are too fat to fit in the scanner or they are claustrophobic. Remember that the patient has to remain motionless for 20–30 minutes to avoid blurred images.

The alternative to an MR scan is a radiculogram that is usually combined with a CT scan (see below). Although a radiculogram is invasive and exposes the patient to a small amount of radiation, it is still sometimes necessary.

Preoperative management

Investigations

If the cause of the back pain is not clinically obvious, then a screen for possible causes should be performed.

This should include the following:

- Chest radiograph.
- Full blood count.
- ESR.
- Urea and electrolytes.
- Blood glucose.
- Liver function tests.
- Calcium and alkaline phosphatase.
- Serum immunoelectrophoresis.
- Radioisotope bone scan.

If there are signs of nerve root compression and surgery is being considered, the diagnosis is confirmed by a MR scan or a CT radiculogram.

Procedure: radiculogram (lumbar myelogram)

A water-soluble radio-opaque 'dye' is injected into the cerebrospinal fluid via a spinal needle. The nerve roots are outlined and compression of the nerves shows up as a filling defect in the column of contrast. A specimen of cerebrospinal fluid is sent to microbiology for microscopy, culture and sensitivity, and to chemical pathology for estimation of the protein content. After the plain films have been taken, a CT scan of the abnormal levels, with the contrast still in place, may reveal additional information.

Indications

- Sciatica and the clinical features suggestive of a prolapsed intervertebral disc.
- Symptoms of spinal stenosis (see Chapter 52).
- Possible spinal tumour.

Contra-indications

- Back pain without leg pain.
- A patient who will not consider surgery even if the radiculogram shows nerve root compression.

Codes

GA/LA	LA
Blood	0
Antibiotics	0
Time	1 hour
Stay	Day case or overnight
Follow-up	10 days
Off work	3 days

Requirements

Since a radiculogram is an invasive procedure with some risks, the patient has to give signed consent. In many hospitals it is the house officer rather than the radiologist who obtains the consent.

Postradiculogram care

Management

The postradiculogram instructions are usually provided by the radiologist. The patient is encouraged to drink fluids, to stay in bed for 12 hours but is allowed to sit up at 30°.

Complications

Postradiculogram headache. If this occurs, rest the patient in bed and prescribe a mild analgesic. The patient should remain in hospital until comfortable enough to go home. Although the headache usually occurs within 24 hours, it can start after the patient has left the hospital and the patient should be warned of this.

Treatment

Conservative treatment

For an acute, severe episode of back pain, including patients who clinically have a prolapsed disc, the initial treatment is always non-operative. Bed rest has been the traditional treatment but has been shown to be no better than early mobilization. Patients are only admitted if they cannot manage at home and have severe pain. For example, if they live alone up several flights of stairs.

You should prescribe a strong analgesic, such as co-proxamol to be taken regularly rather than p.r.n. Ensure that the patient does not become constipated – back pain and constipation are an unpleasant combination. Also, prescribe a non-steroidal anti-inflammatory.

As soon as the severe symptoms diminish, the patient should be encouraged to mobilize with the help of the physiotherapist.

Remember that 90% of patients with back pain will improve without any major intervention.

Indications for surgery
The patient may be helped by a epidural injection of steroid if they have:
- Back pain and sciatica, but the MR scan that does not correlate with the clinical findings.
- Back pain and sciatica that does correlate with the MR scan.
- Persistent leg pain following disc surgery.

Epidural injections are often performed by the anaesthetist in the Pain Clinic.

Disc excision and nerve root decompression is indicated for the patient with all the following:
- Severe leg pain that has not improved after several weeks of conservative treatment.
- A disc prolapse that is proven on a CT radiculogram or MR scan.
- Clinical features which are consistent with the abnormal level of the radiological investigations.

Contra-indications to surgery
- Back pain with minimal leg pain.
- Improving symptoms.

Procedure: caudal or lumbar epidural steroid injection

A cocktail of local anaesthetic, steroid and saline is introduced into the epidural space. The injection is either via the sacral hiatus – a caudal epidural or a direct lumbar epidural. The success rate is only 70% and it may take some weeks before there is any improvement.

Codes

GA/LA	GA
Blood	0
Antibiotics	0
Time	15 minutes
Drains	0
Plaster	0
Postoperative radiograph	0
Stay	Day case
Follow-up	12 weeks
Off work	2 days

Requirements

The injection can be performed in the anaesthetic room.

Post-procedure care

The patient may become hypotensive in the first few hours after the epidural injection. If this occurs elevate the foot of the bed and prescribe intravenous fluid.

The patient should commence back exercises immediately.

Complications

- Hypotension.
- Acute retention of urine.
- No improvement in symptoms.

Operation: excision of prolapsed intervertebral disc (discectomy/fenestration/laminectomy/microdiscectomy)

The extradural space is entered through a midline posterior incision. Generally only the ligamentum flavum needs to be removed, but if this gives an insufficient view, part of the lamina is removed – a fenestration. In the past, the whole lamina was removed, hence the operation was known as a laminectomy. If the operating microscope is used, the incision is considerably smaller and the operation is known as a micro-discectomy.

If the disc is actually prolapsed, the pieces that lie outside the annulus but under the posterior longitudinal ligament are removed. If the disc is bulging without having prolapsed completely, the posterior ligament and the annular ligament are incised and the disc material removed from the disc space. This is a little hazardous, as the anterior relation to the anterior longitudinal ligament is the aorta. There have been (rare) cases where a hole has been made in the aorta, with fatal consequences!

The patient must be aware that the aim of the operation is to remove leg pain and prevent permanent neurological deficit in the leg. The aim is not to cure the back pain, which may remain postoperatively.

Codes

GA/LA	GA
Blood	Group and save
Antibiotics	Yes
Time	1.5 hours
Drains	0
Plaster	0
Postoperative radiograph	0
Stay	5 days
Follow-up	6 weeks
Off work	2–3 months

Operative requirements

The patient is generally operated upon in the prone position. However, some surgeons prefer the patient to be in the lateral position with the side to be explored uppermost. This does have the advantage that blood runs out of the wound, rather than pooling at the bottom.

For a micro-discectomy, the image intensifier is used to ascertain the correct level prior to making the skin incision. For a non micro-discectomy, a plain radiograph is occasionally taken to check the level. Ask the surgeon if this is his practice, so that you can arrange for the radiographer to be in theatre.

Postoperative care

Management

The house officer must check that the patient is neurologically intact immediately postoperatively.

Mobilization regimes vary from surgeon to surgeon. When the patient can arch their back and perform a straight-leg raise, they can get out of bed and be mobilized with the help of the physiotherapist.

No heavy lifting for at least 6 months.

Complications

- Temporary or permanent damage of the nerve root can occur. This would give an isolated muscle group and dermatome deficit – not paraplegia as many patients imagine.
- Dural tear – if this is not sealed at operation, a persistent leak can lead to the formation of a CSF fistula.
- Extradural haematoma – this gives a cauda equina syndrome and requires urgent decompression.
- Wound infection.
- Persisting leg pain.
- Discitis – infection in the disc space.
- Operating on the wrong level, leading to persistent symptoms and further surgery at the correct level.
- Spinal instability.

52 Spinal stenosis

The condition

Spinal stenosis is narrowing of the bony spinal canal resulting in compression of the nerves within the bony canal. It may be due to hypertrophy of the posterior disc margin, osteophytes on the facet joints and/or infolding of the ligamentum flavum. The stenosis may also be due to a degenerative spondylolisthesis. This is a slippage forward of one vertebra on the one below, with resultant narrowing of the bony canal. The bony canal may be congenitally narrow as in achondroplastic dwarfs.

Making the diagnosis

The patient
The patient is usually elderly.

The history
The patient complains of pain and/or heaviness in both legs or occasionally only one leg. The patient may describe the pain as a cramp in the calf muscles. The pain may only occur during exercise. The patient may know how far they can walk before the pain comes on. The pain diminishes when the patient rests with the spine flexed, e.g. leaning forwards. This history is very similar to that of vascular claudication.

On examination
A full general examination should be performed.

A complete neurological examination of the lower limbs must be performed. Look for signs of nerve root irritation. You may be able to reproduce the symptoms by exercising the patient. An ankle jerk that was present prior to the exercise, may be absent after exercise.

Check that the lower limb pulses are present to exclude a true vascular cause for the symptoms.

Radiographs

The lateral view of the lumbosacral spine will show a spondylolisthesis if present.

A CT radiculogram or an MR scan will demonstrate the reduced cross-sectional area of the bony spinal canal. The stenosis is commonly confined to a short segment of spinal canal. You can usually see the hypertrophied ligamentum flavum. The cauda equina may be squashed into a triangular shape.

Treatment

Indications for surgery

Severe symptoms and radiological confirmation of spinal stenosis.

Operation: decompression of spinal stenosis

We make a midline posterior incision. The bone and ligament that are compressing the dura are excised. The number of levels that are decompressed depends on the findings on the CT radiculogram or MR scan. If, after an extensive decompression, the surgeon feels that the spine may potentially be unstable, an intertransverse fusion is performed at the same time. Bone graft is taken from the iliac crest. Some surgeons use internal fixation to stabilize the fusion.

Codes

GA/LA	GA
Blood	Group and save
Antibiotics	Optional
Time	1.5 hours
Drains	0
Plaster	0
Postoperative radiograph	0
Stay	10 days
Follow-up	6 weeks
Off work	3 months

Operative requirements

The patient is operated upon in the prone position. If an intertransverse fusion is planned at the same operation as the decompression, you must note on the consent and the theatre list that a posterior iliac crest bone graft is to be taken.

Postoperative care

Management

The patient is mobilized as comfort allows.

Elderly patients often suffer urinary retention. If a urethral catheter is inserted, it should be left in place until the patient is mobile.

A reflex ileus is common, so ensure that bowel sounds are present before allowing the patient to eat and drink.

If there has been a dural tear, the patient should be kept on bed rest for 2–3 weeks to try to prevent fistula formation.

Complications

- Urinary retention.
- Paralytic ileus.
- Wound infection.
- Persistent leg pain.
- Discitis – infection in the disc space.
- Temporary or permanent damage of the nerve root. This is a rare complication. This would only give weakness in an isolated muscle group and numbness in a single dermatome – not paraplegia as many patients imagine.
- Dural tear – if this is not sealed at operation, a persistent leak can lead to the formation of a CSF fistula.
- Extradural haematoma – this gives a cauda equina syndrome and requires urgent decompression.

Back pain associated with spinal instability

The condition

The most common type of instability is a spondylolisthesis. This is a forward slip of the vertebra above on the one below. The 'instability' is not such that sudden movement occurs between adjacent vertebrae. The abnormal movement occurs insidiously. A spondylolisthesis may be secondary to:

1. Spondylolysis – a defect in the pars interarticularis that may be familial or the result of a stress fracture.
2. Spondylosis – degenerative changes in the facet joints.
3. Postoperative instability following an extensive laminectomy.

Excessive movement between adjacent vertebrae as the patient flexes and extends can also cause pain.

A previous fracture of a vertebral body may result in damage to the intervertebral disc that gives rise to pain.

Making the diagnosis

The history

The patient may have had previous surgery to the spine or an injury. The patient complains of back pain that is well localized. The pain is usually intermittent, coming on after exercise. Take a full history that includes the duration, nature, site, radiation and exacerbating factors of the pain. Ask about bowel and bladder function.

On examination

Perform a complete neurological examination of the lower limbs that should include the following tests:

(a) ask the patient to heel walk and toe walk, this demonstrates muscle weakness (or lack of it) around the ankle;

(b) compare the straight-leg raise with the patient sitting on the edge of the bed and lifting each leg in turn, with the straight-leg raise with the patient lying flat. Inconsistency between the two examinations of the straight-leg raise may be an indicator of psychological overlay. Always include a rectal examination.

Radiographs

Order AP and lateral views of the lumbo-sacral spine. If abnormal movement between the adjacent vertebrae is suspected ask for lateral views in flexion and extension.

If there is a spondylolisthesis due to a spondylolysis, oblique views of the lumbar spine may be needed to show the bony defect of the pars interarticularis. If nerve root involvement has to be excluded, a CT radiculogram or an MR scan are usually required.

Treatment

Indications for surgery

Persistent back pain with a progressive slip, instability or disc damage.

Operation: intertransverse fusion/alar-transverse fusion

We either make a single midline posterior incision, two separate parallel paravertebral vertical incisions, or a single horizontal incision. The spinal canal is not exposed unless the fusion accompanies a spinal decompression. Cancellous bone for grafting is taken from the posterior iliac crest. The transverse processes are exposed and decorticated. Bone graft is laid upon the transverse processes and the gap in between. The facet joints have their articular cartilage removed and then bone graft is inserted into the joints to fuse them.

If the fusion is between adjacent lumbar vertebrae it is termed 'intertransverse'. If the fusion is between the transverse processes of L5 and the ala of the sacrum, it is called an alar-transverse fusion.

Codes

GA/LA	GA
Blood	2 units
Antibiotics	0

Time	1.5 hours
Drains	Yes
Plaster	(Rarely) hip spica
Postoperative radiograph	0
Stay	10 days
Follow-up	6 weeks
Off work	2–3 months, depending on occupation

Postoperative care

Management
The patient stays on bed rest until he is able to bridge (i.e. arch the back).

Urinary retention is common postoperatively. If a catheter is inserted, it should be left in until the patient is able to get out of bed. However, you must ensure that the retention is not neurologically based, by checking that the patient has the feeling of a full bladder and has normal perianal sensation and rectal tone.

A reflex ileus is common, so ensure that bowel sounds are present before allowing the patient to eat and drink.

The patient may be immobilized in a plaster hip spica but this is not common. If used, the plaster is applied after 5 days postoperatively and is kept on for 5 weeks.

Complications
- Urinary retention.
- Deep vein thrombosis.
- Failure of fusion.
- Persistence of back pain, even if the fusion is solid.
- Persistent pain from the iliac crest bone graft donor site.

CHAPTER 54

Vertebral crush fracture

The condition

A vertebral crush fracture results from a mainly vertical force going up the spine. The vertebrae at the thoraco-lumbar junction are the most commonly fractured. The first lumbar vertebra is the most common level of a crush fracture.

In young adults, considerable force is required to fracture a vertebra. The bone is more resistant to compression than in the elderly, so the vertebra tends to spread. Fragments of bone may intrude into the spinal canal. These may press on the spinal cord and give neurological problems. However, surprisingly large fragments of bone may lie in the canal without any clinical neurological deficit.

In the elderly osteoporotic female, a crush fracture may result from a trivial fall. In the elderly it is almost always a stable injury.

Making the diagnosis

The history

In the young, there is a history of a fall from a height with the patient landing either on their feet or their backside. Alternatively the patient may have been in a car accident. The patient has severe pain at the level of the crushed vertebra. He may have other fractures. If he has had a fall you should ask about heel pain in particular.

The elderly patient will have a history of a stumble or gentle fall. However the pain may be quite severe and may be enough to incapacitate the patient so that admission to hospital is necessary.

Ask about bowel and bladder function.

On examination

Log roll the patient (with help from the nurses) and examine the back. Identify the level of maximal tenderness and look for a gibbus (a prominence due to a forward angulation in the spinal column).

Perform a rectal examination.

Perform a full neurological examination of lower limbs.

Radiographs

Obtain good quality AP and lateral views of the lumbar spine. If there are doubts about the stability of the spine, a CT scan is required.

Initial management

Treat the patient as if they have an unstable fracture until definitely disproved. This means log rolling the patient in order to turn them, and avoiding flexion and extension.

Preoperative management

Common associated injuries

Calcaneal fractures.

Treatment

For elderly patients, all that is required is for the patient to be on bed rest for a few days while the pain settles. They are then gently mobilized in a corset with the help of the physiotherapists.

In the younger patient who has no abnormal neurological findings and an anterior compression that is less than 50% of the height of the vertebral body, treatment consists of bed rest for 6 weeks, followed by mobilization in a plaster or plastic jacket.

Indications for surgery

An unstable fracture.

A fracture with fragments of bone in the spinal canal (seen on the CT scan) and a deteriorating neurological deficit.

Young patients with greater than 50% loss of vertebral height.

Operation: decompression of the spinal canal and Harrington rod stabilization

The spine is approached posteriorly. If indicated, the bony canal is opened and the bone fragments removed.

Harrington rods with sublaminal hooks are used to distract and thus reduce the fracture. One rod is placed on each side of the spinous processes and they are attached to broad hooks that are slipped under the edges of the laminae. The instrumentation is fixed to the two vertebra above and the two below the vertebra that is fractured.

Codes

GA/LA	GA
Blood	4 units
Antibiotics	Yes
Time	2 hours
Drains	Yes
Plaster	0
DVT prophylaxis	Yes
Postoperative radiograph	AP and lateral lumbar spine
Stay	2 weeks
Follow-up	6 weeks
Off work	3 months

Postoperative care

Management
Once the spine has been stabilized, the patient is safe to be mobilized as the pain allows. Urinary catheterization is often required postoperatively.

Complications
- Neural damage that may include making an incomplete neurological lesion complete.
- Infection.
- Late pull out of a sublaminal hook.

55

Pelvic fracture (excluding pubic rami fracture of the elderly)

The condition

Considerable energy is required for a pelvis to fracture. This injury is usually part of a multiple injury.

Pelvic fractures can result in secondary rupture of the venous plexus in the pelvis that in turn leads to massive internal haemorrhage. Remember that a patient with a displaced pelvic fracture can exsanguinate without a drop of blood being lost onto the bed!

Making the diagnosis

The history

One needs to know the exact mechanism of injury. If the patient was in a road traffic accident, was he/she the driver of the vehicle? Was he/she wearing a seat belt? At what speed did the impact occur?

Take a history that does not concentrate on the obvious injury. You need to know about the patient's general health, etc. You also need to know where else he hurts.

Ask the patient or the attendants if the patient has passed urine spontaneously since the injury.

On examination

Examine the whole patient, as the force required to fracture a pelvis can damage other bones or viscera.

Examine the perineum for bruising.

Look for blood at the urethral meatus that may signify a urethral injury.

Note the leg lengths. If one leg is shortened, this is likely to be due to a hip dislocation.

Examine the neuro-vascular status of the lower limbs. Loss of an ankle jerk may be due to sciatic nerve damage.

Radiographs

An AP view of the pelvis is the only view that should be obtained in the resuscitation room.

If the fracture involves the acetabulum, ask for Judet views (iliac and obturator obliques). These show the anterior and posterior columns of the acetabulum. Judet views are not required urgently and can be obtained once the patient is stable.

The pelvis is a ring. If there is a fracture that is displaced, there must be another discontinuity in the ring. Always remember to look at the sacro-iliac joints to see if they are intact.

A CT scan of the pelvis is often required to determine the exact configuration of the fracture. If a hip dislocation has been reduced, a CT scan will show whether or not fragments of bone remain in the joint or if there is a femoral head fracture.

Preoperative management

Investigations

- Full blood count.
- Urinalysis for haematuria.

Common associated injuries

Cervical spine injury, long bone fracture, ruptured urethra, torn bladder and abdominal injury.

Treatment

Emergency treatment

Patients with a pelvic fracture bleed internally, so make sure that there is adequate venous access (two 14 gauge cannulae) and adequate fluid and blood replacement (6 units minimum).

If the patient has not passed urine, consider the possibility that there is a urethral injury. Gently try to pass a urethral catheter. Do not use force, as there is the risk of making an incomplete urethral tear complete. If you experience any difficulty, insert a suprapubic catheter.

If the hip is dislocated, it must be reduced under a general anaesthetic and a femoral traction pin inserted.

If the fracture involves the acetabulum or there is gross displacement of one side of the pelvis, a femoral traction pin should be inserted in the casualty department, using local anaesthetic.

If the pelvic fracture is of the open-book type, the application of an external fixator and closure of the 'book' may help reduce the blood loss.

Definitive treatment

A patient with an undisplaced extra-articular fracture is treated with bed rest for 6 weeks.

An extra-articular pelvic fracture that is unstable needs to be stabilized, either with an external fixator or by open reduction and internal fixation.

Undisplaced and minimally displaced acetabular fractures are usually treated with skeletal traction.

Displaced acetabular fractures need accurate reduction, stable internal fixation and early motion.

Operation: acetabular fracture; insertion of a femoral Denham or Steinmann pin for skeletal traction +/ − manipulation under anaesthesia of dislocated hip

If the hip is dislocated posteriorly, as is common, it is reduced by one person pressing down on both anterior superior iliac spines, while a second person flexes the hip to 90° and then pulls up on the leg.

A Denham pin (which is threaded in its mid part) or a Steinmann pin (which is smooth) is inserted across the distal femur and 6.75 kg (15 lb) of traction is added.

Codes

GA/LA	GA or LA if pin insertion alone
Blood	6 units
Antibiotics	0
Time	30 minutes
Drains	0
Plaster	0
Postoperative radiograph	AP pelvis and Judet views

Stay	6 weeks
Follow-up	6 weeks
Off work	3 months minimum

Operative requirements

Steinmann/Denham pin insertion pack. If the hip needs to be reduced, one or two strong assistants are of great help.

Postoperative care

Management

- Apply 6.75 kg (15 lb) of skeletal traction.
- Monitor the pulse, blood pressure and urine output at least hourly for the first 24 hours.

Complications

- Exsanguination!
- Hip dislocation.
- Urethral injury.
- Associated intra-abdominal injury, e.g. splenic rupture.

Fracture of the pubic rami

The condition

A fractured pubic ramus is a common minor injury in the elderly.

In a younger patient, a pubic ramus fracture is a serious injury and must be treated as a major pelvic fracture (see Chapter 55).

Making the diagnosis

The history
The typical story is of an elderly woman who has suffered a minor fall. She presents present with pain in the hip and is unable to weight bear. The history often leads one to initially suspect that the patient has a fracture of the femoral neck.

On examination
The leg is not short or externally rotated. Examining the movements of the hip may cause some discomfort, but not as much as you find in a patient with a femoral neck fracture.

Radiographs
An AP of the pelvis may show a fracture of one or both pubic rami. If a patient has a lot of hip pain and the radiograph looks normal, order a bone scan. The scan will be hot at the fracture site. The scan will confirm the clinical diagnosis of a pubic ramus fracture that cannot be seen on the radiographs.

Preoperative management

Common associated injuries
Any fracture associated with osteoporosis.

Treatment

The patient is admitted for bed rest and should be prescribed oral analgesia. The patient is helped to mobilize as the pain settles.

Codes

Blood	0
Plaster	0
Stay	10–14 days
Follow-up	6 weeks
DVT prophylaxis	Yes

Complications

Those of an elderly patient confined to bed, i.e. deep vein thrombosis, urinary tract infection, pressure sores, respiratory tract infection.

Lower Limb

Congenital dislocation of the hip

The condition

The incidence of congenital dislocation of the hip is 2.5 per 1000 live births. Dislocation is more common in girls. The left hip is more often affected than the right.

The risk factors are:

- A family history of congenital dislocation of the hip.
- Breech delivery.
- The presence of a foot deformity.
- Any other congenital abnormality.

Making the diagnosis

The patient

A dislocatable or dislocated hip may be diagnosed when the newborn baby is examined for this and other disorders.

Alternatively, the diagnosis may not be made until the child begins to walk and a limp is noticed.

On examination

Place the baby prone on the couch. Look at the skin creases below the buttocks. When a hip is dislocated (as opposed to dislocatable) the creases are asymmetrical. The affected leg is slightly short.

Abduction of the affected leg is restricted. In a normal newborn baby, the flexed hips can be abducted so that the knees touch the couch.

Ortolani's test is positive if there is a palpable clunk when the hip is abducted. The clunk is due to the dislocated hip going back into the socket.

Barlow's test is positive if downward pressure along the femur, with some lateral force, makes a reduced hip dislocate.

In the older child with a dislocated hip, Trendelenburg's sign is positive and there is a Trendelenburg gait.

Radiographs

Radiographs before the child is 6 weeks old are of little value as the head of the femur has not ossified and cannot be seen. After the head begins to ossify, but before it has done so completely, dislocation is inferred by abnormalities in lines drawn onto the AP view of the pelvis.

Preoperative management

Investigations

Ultrasound of the hip is the best way of identifying abnormal hips in the newborn. The advantage is that structures that are not visible on a plain radiograph can be identified. The accuracy of the examination depends on the skill and experience of the ultrasonographer.

An arthrogram of the hip gives information about the congruence of the hip that is easier to interpret than an ultrasound. Radio-opaque contrast is injected into the hip joint and is seen with the image intensifier. Unlike an ultrasound, an arthrogram has to be performed under a general anaesthetic.

Treatment

A newborn with a dislocatable hip, or a hip that is dislocated but can be reduced, is nursed in double nappies or an abduction harness for 6 weeks. The majority of these hips are normal at their 6-week review.

A baby with a dislocated hip that cannot be reduced by Ortolani's test, is placed in gallows traction (legs suspended vertically in skin traction). The legs are gradually abducted to full abduction over 2 weeks. If, with the hips fully abducted, the hip is fully located, the child is placed in a plaster cast that includes both hips. The cast is kept on for 6 weeks. The child is then kept in a splint that prevents adduction but allows some flexion, for a further 10 months.

If, after gradual abduction in gallows traction, the hip remains dislocated, an open reduction is performed.

At open reduction the hip may only be stable with the femur in internal rotation and abduction. If so, the child is placed in a plaster with the leg in the appropriate position for 6 weeks. Then an upper femoral osteotomy is performed to maintain the reduction.

Indications for surgery
A child who is less than 6 years old with a dislocated hip that cannot be reduced by conservative methods.

Operation: open reduction of congenital dislocation of the hip

The hip is approached via an anterior incision. The structures preventing reduction of the hip are removed from the joint and the hip is reduced.

Codes

GA/LA	GA
Blood	Group and save
Antibiotics	0
Time	1.5 hours
Drains	0
Plaster	Hip spica
Postoperative radiograph	AP pelvis
Stay	5 days
Follow-up	6 weeks

Operative requirements
An on-table arthrogram is usually performed prior to open reduction. Theatres and the radiographer need to be informed of this beforehand.

Postoperative care

Management
The hip spica cast is kept on for 6 weeks. If necessary, an upper femoral osteotomy is then performed.

Complication
Avascular necrosis of the femoral head.

Operation: upper femoral osteotomy in a child

The child is placed on an ordinary operating table with a sand-bag under the hip. A lateral incision is made. The upper femur and anterior femoral neck are exposed and the femur is divided. The femur is fixed in the corrected position with a nail plate.

Indications for surgery
This operation has several indications:

- Following open reduction of a congenitally dislocated hip.
- Acetabular dysplasia, with 'uncovering' of the femoral head.
- Excessive femoral neck anteversion resulting in intoeing.

Codes

GA/LA	GA
Blood	Group and save
Antibiotics	Yes
Time	1.5 hours
Drains	0
Plaster	0
Postoperative radiograph	AP pelvis and lateral hip
Stay	7 days
Follow-up	6 weeks
Off school	3–6 weeks

Operative requirements
Check with the surgeon and then specify on the operating list, what type of nail plate is to be used.

A radiolucent operating table should be used, in case an intraoperative check radiograph is necessary.

Postoperative care

Management
The child is allowed out of bed using crutches when the immediate postoperative pain has settled. It is impossible to restrict a child's weight bearing and they should be allowed to do whatever is comfortable.

The plate and screws are removed after 1 year.

Complications
- Wound infection.
- Incorrect orientation of osteotomy.

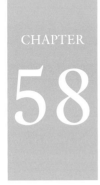

The irritable hip

The condition

This is a nonspecific condition that affects young children. Its significance is that serious causes of hip pain have to be excluded before making the diagnosis of an irritable hip. One must exclude septic arthritis, Perthes' disease, slipped upper femoral epiphysis and tuberculosis.

Making the diagnosis

The patient
The child is usually aged between 4 and 9 years old and will have had no previous hip complaints.

The history
The child complains of an increasing pain in the hip and is unwilling to walk. There may be a history of the child having recently had a cold or flu.

On examination
The child is otherwise well, without a fever. The child will either have a limp or simply refuse to walk. On examination of the hip, all movements will be painful, but the discomfort is worst at the extremes of movement. Extension of the hip is normally the movement that is most severely restricted (and the last to be regained). The child therefore rests with the hip held in flexion.

Radiographs
One must obtain a radiograph of the hip to exclude infection, Perthes' disease and slipped upper femoral epiphysis. By definition, the radiograph is normal in an irritable hip.

Management

Investigations

Blood must be taken for a full blood count, C reactive protein and ery-throcyte sedimentation rate. If the child is very young and you are not practised at drawing blood from children, ask the paediatricians for their help.

Consider obtaining a Heaf test and a chest radiograph if the child is from a community where tuberculosis is common.

Order an ultrasound of the hip. A good ultrasonographer will be able to distinguish a joint effusion from a septic arthritis. There is commonly a small effusion within the hip joint if the child has an irritable hip.

Treatment

Most surgeons prefer to admit a child who is unable or unwilling to weight bear. The child is placed on bed rest, with 2.25 kg (5 lb) of skin traction on the affected leg. After 4 or 5 days, the child should be more comfortable and may be allowed up. Keep the child in hospital until they are completely recovered with a full, pain-free, range of movement. Occasionally, if the surgeon is convinced that the diagnosis is only an irritable hip and the parents are sensible, the child is allowed to rest at home.

The child must be followed up in the clinic for at least 3 months. Radiographs should be taken. This is in case the irritable hip was a preliminary to the development of Perthes' disease.

CHAPTER
59
Slipped upper femoral epiphysis

The condition

The epiphysis of the femoral head can 'slip' off the neck. This may be a gradual or a sudden process. Although it is not common, it is imperative that the condition is diagnosed promptly to prevent the head slipping further than it already has.

Making the diagnosis

The patient

The patient is usually between 10 and 15 years old. Slipped epiphysis is more common in boys. The patient is typically overweight with poor secondary sexual development. The child may have a demonstrable hormone imbalance or deficiency, such as hypothyroidism, but this is rare.

The history

A history of specific trauma is rare. The child may complain of increasing hip pain but often the pain may be referred to the knee. (*Beware the 10-year-old boy with knee pain – examine the hip!*) If the slip is acute-on-chronic, there will a history of mild hip pain that suddenly becomes worse.

On examination

The patient often has a limp. If the femoral head has slipped a lot, the leg will be short and externally rotated. All movements of the hip may be uncomfortable, but the most significant signs are limited internal rotation and limited abduction.

Radiographs

Most slips are visible on an AP view of the pelvis. Compare the normal side to the painful side.

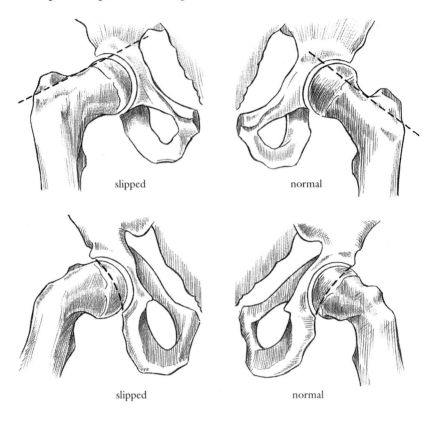

slipped   normal

slipped   normal

A line drawn up the superior edge of the neck of the femur should pass into the head of the femur. If the line passes outside the head, the head has slipped.

The posterior edge of the acetabulum should cut across the medial corner of the upper femoral metaphysis. It does not do so when the epiphysis has slipped.

If there is any doubt about whether or not the epiphysis has slipped on the AP view, ask for frog lateral views of both hips.

Preoperative management

Investigations
Consider hypothyroidism.

Preparation for surgery
While waiting for surgery, the child may be more comfortable with
2.25 kg (5 lb) of skin traction on the affected leg.

Treatment

Indications for surgery
All slipped upper femoral epiphyses require fixation in situ.

Even a severe slip should not be manipulated into a better position
prior to fixation. This is because the manipulation may further damage
the already injured blood supply to the femoral head, resulting in
avascular necrosis.

There is debate whether or not to prophylactically pin the contralateral hip, as bilateral slippage is common (25%). Some surgeons prefer
to instruct the parents to bring in the child at the first sign of any symptoms. Their argument is that the second slip will be diagnosed when
very minor and a procedure on a normal hip may be avoided.

Operation: internal fixation of slipped upper femoral epiphysis

The child is placed on the orthopaedic table in a similar position to an
adult undergoing a DHS. No attempt is made to reduce the head back
into place. Nevertheless, the head may partly reduce purely by positioning the child on the traction table. A small lateral incision is made
down to the greater trochanter. Guide wires are inserted up the femoral
neck into the femoral head. The position of the guide wires is checked
with the image intensifier. Cannulated screws are passed over the guide
wires. The number of screws used varies depending on the child, the
amount of slippage of the femoral head and the surgeon. With a severe
slip, the head may be so far backwards that the entry point for the
screws may be quite anterior on the neck.

Codes
GA/LA	GA
Blood	Group and save
Antibiotics	Yes

Time	1 hour
Drains	0
Plaster	0
Postoperative radiograph	AP pelvis and lateral hip
Stay	1 week
Follow-up	6 weeks
Off school	4 weeks

Operative requirements

The requirements are the same as when inserting a dynamic hip screw, i.e. image intensifier and radiographer.

The surgeon should specify the type of implant to be used.

Postoperative care

Management

- Full blood count at 48 hours.
- Encourage the child to mobilize the hip and knee while in bed.
- When the pain subsides the child is allowed up, non-weight-bearing with crutches.

Complications

- Poor fixation leading to further slippage.
- Attempted reduction can lead to avascular necrosis of the femoral head.
- Penetration of the pin through the articular cartilage of the femoral head may cause pain on movement of the hip and damage to the articular cartilage.

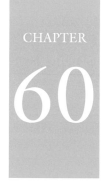

Arthritis of the hip

The condition

Osteoarthritis of the hip may be primary, or secondary to trauma or to previous joint disease.

Rheumatoid arthritis frequently results in the destruction of the hip joints.

Making the diagnosis

The patient

A patient who presents for a joint replacement is usually over 60 years, but not always. Patients with rheumatoid arthritis may be much younger.

The history

Ask about predisposing factors including family history, hip problems as a child (sepsis, congenital dislocation of the hip, Perthes' disease and slipped upper femoral capital epiphysis) and trauma. Ask the patient if they have pain coming from other joints. If the patient has rheumatoid arthritis, it is important to know which joint is causing the most distress. Ask the patient if he has any back pain. Often back problems can give pain that radiates to the hip and leg that may confuse the clinical picture.

When taking the specific history of the hip pain, you should establish:

- The severity and any radiation of the pain.
- Whether or not the pain wakes the patient at night.
- What analgesics the patient takes and how often.
- Whether or not the patient is able to put his shoes and socks on normally.
- Whether or not the patient is able to cut his own toe nails.

- How the patient goes up stairs? Normally, or by placing both feet on each step, holding onto the bannister?
- If the patient uses a stick indoors or just outdoors.
- Whether or not the patient has a limp.

Take a social history that includes the patient's occupation, hobbies, home circumstances. Does he live in a flat or a house with stairs? Does the patient live alone?

On examination
Watch the patient walk. Note any limp and if he uses a stick.

Look for scars from previous operations around the hip. Perform Trendelenburg's test to test for weak abductors. Note any fixed flexion deformity with Thomas's test. (If you do not know how to perform these tests, ask your Consultant to show you.)

Examine the range of flexion, abduction and adduction of both hips. Examine external and internal rotation with the hips extended.

- Look for apparent shortening and measure true shortening.
- Check that the foot pulses are present.
- Check that there are no abnormal neurological findings in the lower limb.
- Do not omit a rectal examination of the prostate from the examination of a male patient.

Radiographs
Ensure that there is a recent AP view of the whole pelvis and a lateral view of the affected hip.

If the patient has rheumatoid arthritis (with neck symptoms), obtain AP and lateral views of the cervical spine to exclude instability.

Preoperative management

Investigations
Midstream urine.

Preparation for surgery
Some surgeons like their patients to have a shower or bath, washing with an antiseptic soap, the night before and on the day of surgery.

Treatment

The initial treatment for all arthritic joints is medical. This includes analgesics and anti-inflammatory drugs, as well as physiotherapy. The use of a walking stick and a non-steroidal anti-inflammatory drug may be enough to relieve the pain of many patients.

Indications for surgery

A total hip replacement is indicated for either osteoarthritis or rheumatoid arthritis of the hip if the patient has severe pain that interferes with his quality of life. Stiffness alone is not an indication for performing a joint replacement.

It is also indicated for failed fixation of a subcapital hip fracture.

A total hip replacement may fail because of either deep infection or loosening. If at all possible, the hip replacement is renewed. However, this may not be possible and the patient may be left with a Girdlestone's excision arthroplasty.

Contra-indications to total hip replacement

Minimal symptoms, however bad the radiographic changes.

Ischaemic heart disease or peripheral vascular disease that would obscure the benefits of hip replacement; i.e. if the angina or claudication is so severe that the patient would still not be able to walk very far following surgery, the risks may outweigh the benefits.

Urinary tract infection.

Prostatism that may result in postoperative urinary retention and the need for a prostatectomy. It is better to have the urological investigations and surgery *before* a total hip replacement.

Operation: total hip replacement

The hip can be approached through a variety of routes. The postero-lateral, the lateral and the antero-lateral are the three common approaches.

Once exposed, we dislocate the hip joint. The acetabulum is prepared by removing the remaining articular cartilage and the hard sclerotic bone. The femoral head and part of the neck are removed and the femoral canal is prepared to take the stem of the component.

Hip replacements generally have a metal femoral stem with a metal head, which articulates with a high density polyethylene acetabular cup. The acetabular component may be totally plastic or may be metal backed.

The components may be held in place with bone cement, methyl-methacrylate. The cement contains barium so we can see it on the radiographs. The cement may also contain an antibiotic. Remember that cement is not a glue and works by its interdigitation rather than adhesion.

Alternatively, one or both components may be inserted 'un-cemented', with the femoral stem being a press fit, and the acetabulum being either a press fit or held by screws or pegs. Lack of cement has the theoretical advantage of making subsequent revision surgery easier, but the disadvantage of having an initially poorer fixation. Uncemented components are often used for younger patients (under 60 years), since the likelihood of needing a revision is high. Some uncemented components are coated with hydroxyapatite. This has a structure that is similar to coral and bone grows into the hydroxyapatite.

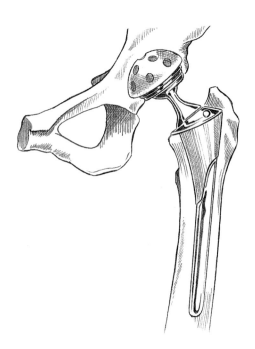

At best, a hip replacement may last 15–20 years, but sometimes it may last less than 5 years.

Codes

GA/LA	GA or spinal
Blood	3 units
Antibiotics	Yes
Time	2 hours
Drains	Yes
Plaster	0
Postoperative radiograph	AP whole pelvis and lateral hip
DVT prophylaxis	Yes
Stay	10 days
Follow-up	6 weeks
Off work	3 months

Operative requirements

State on the operating list exactly what prosthesis is to be used and whether or not it is inserted with cement.

Postoperative care

Management

Check and document that the femoral nerve and the sciatic nerve are intact. Ask the patient to press their knee into the bed. If the quadriceps tighten, the femoral nerve is intact. If the patient can wiggle their toes and has sensation in the foot, the sciatic nerve is undamaged.

Remove the drains after 24 hours.

Check haemoglobin on postoperative day 2.

If the patient does not pass urine and has to be catheterized, you must give him/her an appropriate antibiotic while the catheter is in place.

The regime for mobilization depends upon the surgical approach and whether the components are cemented or uncemented:

(a) If uncemented components have been implanted, the patient is usually kept partial weight-bearing with crutches for 2–3 months. If both components are cemented the patient can fully weight bear immediately.

(b) The posterior approach to the hip requires that the patient should avoid sitting up for 3–5 days. During this time the patient should go straight from bed to standing. Anterior and lateral approaches to the hip are more stable with the hip flexed than the posterior approach and so the patient can sit in a chair immediately.

(c) Since the posterior approach is potentially unstable in adduction and internal rotation, the patient's locker is kept on the same side of the bed as the operated leg and the patient is advised to sleep on his back for 6 weeks following surgery. This is because, as the patient rolls onto their side, the upper leg falls into adduction and internal rotation, whereas the lower leg stays in neutral. If the patient cannot tolerate sleeping on their back, then they may sleep on the operated side with a pillow between the legs.

Many patients ask about when they can be allowed to drive:

(a) A patient will usually regain their preoperative reaction time by 2 months postoperatively and is then safe to drive.

(b) If they drive an automatic car and the left leg has been operated upon, they can drive sooner than if it was the right leg.

(c) It is the patient's ultimate decision whether or not they feel safe to drive.

Complications

- Injury to nerves and vessels.
- Intraoperative femur fracture.
- Wound infection.
- Deep vein thrombosis and pulmonary embolism.
- Loosening of one or both components.
- Infection of the prosthesis.

Operation: revision of total hip replacement

This is a considerably more difficult operation than a primary hip replacement. The exposure has to be more extensive and the soft tissue dissection greater.

If loose, removal of the components themselves is easy. However, removal of the bone cement from the femoral shaft can be a painstaking and laborious task. As the cortex is often thinner than normal, there is the dual risk of either perforating the shaft and/or breaking it. Special cement-removing equipment is needed and a special revision prosthesis may be required. Autogenous or banked bone may be needed to fill defects.

If the original prosthesis is being removed for infection, the revision is usually performed in two stages. At the first operation, the infected components are removed, samples of tissue and fluid are sent for microbiological examination and beads containing an antibiotic are left in the wound. The second operation is performed after 6 weeks treatment with the appropriate antibiotics, when the new prosthesis is inserted.

Codes

GA/LA	GA
Blood	6 units
Antibiotics	Yes
Time	2–4 hours
Drains	Yes
Plaster	0
Postoperative radiograph	AP pelvis and lateral hip
DVT prophylaxis	Yes
Stay	2 weeks
Follow-up	6 weeks
Off work	3 months

Operative requirements

Cement-removing instruments.

The theatre list should state if one or both components are to be revised, what design/make is being removed and what type is going to be inserted.

If only one component is to be removed, the femoral head must be of the same circumference as the inner diameter of the acetabular cup, so look in the notes to see what size was originally used. Common head sizes are 22 mm, 28 mm and 32 mm.

If a long-stemmed femoral component is anticipated as being necessary, ensure that it is available.

Postoperative care

Management

The intraoperative and postoperative blood loss can be considerable. You must check the amount of drainage in recovery on the evening of the first day post operation, and the next morning. The amount of blood replaced should nearly equal the amount of total blood lost.

Check that the femoral nerve and the sciatic nerve are intact. Ask the patient to press their knee into the bed. If the quadriceps tighten, the femoral nerve is intact. If the patient can wiggle their toes and has sensation in the foot, the sciatic nerve is undamaged.

If the arthroplasty seemed a little unstable on the operating table, the patient may need to remain on bed rest for longer than usual or may even require skeletal traction.

Due to the greater tissue dissection, patients who have had a revision hip take longer to mobilize than after a primary total hip replacement. Otherwise, the mobilization instructions are similar to those given for a primary hip replacement.

Complications

The complications associated with primary hip surgery are all more common after revision surgery:
- Injury to nerves and vessels.
- Intraoperative femoral fracture.
- Dislocation.
- Deep vein thrombosis and pulmonary embolism.
- Infection of the prosthesis.
- Loosening of one or other components.

CHAPTER 61

Dislocated total hip replacement

The condition

A total hip replacement is most at risk of dislocating in the immediate postoperative period. This commences with the patient being moved off the operating table onto their bed. In the first days and weeks, the muscles are weak and there is no scar tissue around the new joint. It is during this time that most care must be taken.

The position in which a total hip replacement is most unstable partly depends on the surgical approach that was used to insert the prosthesis. The patient should be instructed to avoid putting their hip into an unstable position.

Following the posterior approach, the hip is most at risk when flexed, adducted and internally rotated.

Following the antero-lateral and the lateral approaches, the hip is most unstable in extension with external rotation.

More than one dislocation may indicate malposition of one or both components and the prosthesis may need to be revised.

A total hip may survive for many years without a problem. It can dislocate due to wear of the acetabular component.

Making the diagnosis

The history

When taking the history, you must find out exactly what the patient was doing and the position of the patient's leg when the hip dislocated, especially if it has occurred more than once.

On examination

If the hip is dislocated posteriorly, the leg lies shortened, slightly flexed and internally rotated. If the dislocation is anterior, the leg lies extended and externally rotated.

231

Radiographs

Ask for an AP pelvis and a lateral view of the hip.

Treatment

If the hip is very unstable, it may be possible to relocate the joint under intravenous sedation on the ward. However, it is usually safer to give the patient a general anaesthetic in the operating theatre.

Operation: reduction of dislocated total hip replacement

The hip is usually easily reduced by a combination of gentle traction and internal or external rotation. One should screen the hip under the image intensifier to find out how easily it dislocates and in what position. The surgeon can then decide on how to manage the patient. For example if the hip is very unstable with the hip extended and in external rotation, the surgeon may decide to apply a below knee plaster with a 'derotation' bar to keep the leg internally rotated.

Codes

GA/LA	GA
Blood	0
Antibiotics	0
Time	10 minutes
Drains	0
Plaster	Occasionally
Postoperative radiograph	AP and lateral hip
Stay	Depends on time since original operation
Follow-up	6 weeks
Off work	6 weeks

Operative requirements

Image intensifier and radiographer.

Postoperative care

Management

If the patient is in the immediate postoperative period, the surgeon may decide to keep the patient on bed rest on traction for 6 weeks to allow the false capsule to form.

If the hip is unstable in flexion, we may put a plaster cylinder on the patient to prevent them from flexing the hip past 90°.

It may be possible to allow the patient to mobilize wearing a hinged brace. This has to be worn for 24 hours a day. The brace can be adjusted to allow movement within a certain range.

Complications

- Recurrent dislocation.
- Inability to reduce the hip closed, necessitating an open reduction.

Fracture of the neck of the femur

The condition

This is a common fracture among the elderly and is due to osteoporosis.

The proportion of elderly in the population is increasing, as is the age-specific incidence of the fracture. This will result in an exponential rise in the overall incidence of this fracture in the next 10–20 years.

Although these fractures are of the neck of the femur, they are commonly referred to as hip fractures.

The anatomical location of the fracture influences the treatment. The main differentiation depends on whether the fracture is intra-capsular or extracapsular.

The main source of blood supply to the femoral head is through the vessels that enter the bone at the base of the neck, at the site of attachment of the capsule. Therefore, intracapsular fractures result in the blood supply to the femoral head being put at risk by being interrupted. If an intracapsular fracture is reduced and internally fixed, the fracture may not unite. Alternatively the fracture may unite but the femoral head may become avascular. The greater the displacement of the fracture, the greater the likelihood of either non-union of the fracture or of avascular necrosis of the femoral head. Although intracapsular fractures can be divided into subcapital, transcervical and basicervical, they are all referred to as subcapital fractures in general parlance.

Extracapsular fractures do not damage the blood supply to the femoral head, and generally unite after reduction and internal fixation.

Patients with a fractured neck of femur are associated with at least 30% mortality in the 6 months following surgery.

Making the diagnosis

The patient
These elderly patients are often infirm and have multiple medical and social problems. It is these problems that usually prevent the patient's speedy return to their pre-injury abode rather than the fracture itself.

The history
There will be a history of either a stumble or of the leg giving way. The patient has pain in the hip that prevents them weight bearing.

A full history must be taken from either the patient or the carer who may accompany the patient into hospital. If there is any doubt about past history or present medications, telephone the patient's general practitioner.

■ Establish the walking ability of the patient prior to the fall.
■ Ask about the patient's home circumstances. Does the patient live alone? If not, how fit is the spouse? Are there stairs up to the front door and/or inside? Does the patient have relatives or friends nearby?

If the patient lives in a nursing home, find out what level of activity is required before they can return to the home.

On examination
The injured leg is typically shortened, externally rotated and painful. Check the neurovascular integrity of the limb, especially the foot pulses.

Radiographs
Request an AP of the pelvis and a lateral view of the painful hip. Intracapsular fractures are graded radiologically according to the Garden classification:

Garden I   Incomplete fracture through one cortex only.
Garden II   Complete fracture running across the neck but without displacement.
Garden III   Complete fracture with partial displacement, with the femoral head adducted relative to the neck.
Garden IV   Complete fracture with full displacement, so that the femoral head is translocated relative to the neck.

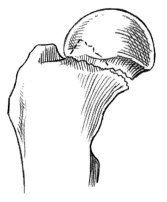

Garden I (impacted)

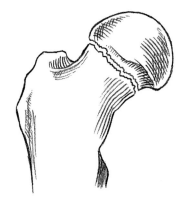

Garden II (undisplaced)

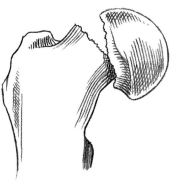

Garden III (rotated)

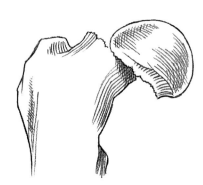

Garden IV (separated)

Preoperative management

Preparation for surgery

Many of the patients spend the night on the floor before being found and they may already be quite dehydrated prior to being kept nil by mouth while waiting for surgery. If there is likely to be a delay in the patient being operated upon, start an intravenous infusion.

The traditional practice is to put 2.25 kg (5 lb) of skin traction on the injured leg. The traction is meant to reduce the patient's pain. However patients are often more uncomfortable in traction, and are better off without any.

Treatment

Patients with a femoral neck fracture are almost always treated by surgery. These fractures are operated upon to allow the patient to mobilize as quickly as possible and to try to avoid the complications of prolonged bed rest in the elderly.

Indications for surgery

Undisplaced or minimally displaced intracapsular (Garden grade I or II) hip fractures are fixed using pins or screws.

Displaced intracapsular fractures are usually reduced and fixed in patients less than 70 years old. Reduction and internal fixation is contraindicated in patients who:

- Are on steroid therapy.
- Have poor mental health.
- Have an interval between fracture and surgery greater than 48 hours.

The benefit of 'saving' the femoral head is in avoiding the complications of a hemiarthroplasty. The complications of a hemiarthroplasty include:

- Pain in the hip, due to articulation of metal on cartilage.
- Dislocation.
- Infection.
- Femoral fracture around the stem.
- Acetabular erosion.

On the other hand, if the fracture unites, there is a 20–30% risk of avascular necrosis of the femoral head, which would then necessitate performing a total hip replacement.

In the older patient with an intracapsular fracture, the head of the femur is replaced by a hemiarthroplasty. The commonest prostheses used are the Austin-Moore, which is inserted without cement, and the Thompson's that is inserted with cement. Some surgeons use a 'bipolar' prosthesis.

Intertrochanteric hip fractures are reduced and then held with a dynamic hip screw, also known as a pin and plate.

Operation: dynamic hip screw for intertrochanteric fracture of the neck of the femur

The patient is placed supine on the orthopaedic traction table with their feet in the traction boots. Ensure that the feet are well padded and

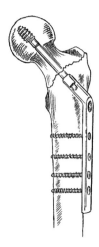

secure. If they are not secure, they will pull out of the boots when traction is applied. The fracture is screened using the image intensifier and is reduced prior to making the incision. We make a straight lateral incision down to the upper femur. A guide wire is passed up the neck of the femur under image intensifier control and the reamer for the screw passed over the guide wire. The large lag screw is inserted up the neck and then the plate and barrel are applied to the femur and held with screws.

As the fracture heals, it collapses. The sliding design of the screw within a barrel allows this to happen without the screw cutting out of the head. This is the 'dynamic' concept.

Codes

GA/LA	GA
Blood	2 units
Antibiotics	Yes
Time	1 hour
Drains	Yes
Plaster	0
Postoperative radiograph	AP pelvis and lateral hip
DVT prophylaxis	Yes
Stay	2 weeks minimum
Follow-up	6 weeks

Operative requirements
- Image intensifier and radiographer.
- Orthopaedic traction table.

Postoperative care

Management
The patient is mobilized, fully weight-bearing, as soon as the drain has been removed.

Check the haemoglobin on the second postoperative day.

Consider the social circumstances of the patient early and refer to social workers or geriatrician if necessary.

Complications
- Wound infection.
- Failure of fixation.
- Chest infection.
- Deep vein thrombosis.
- Urinary tract infection.
- Pressure sores.

Operation: internal fixation of subcapital fracture of the neck of the femur

The patient is placed supine on the orthopaedic traction table with the feet held in the traction boots. Ensure that the feet are well padded and secure. The fracture is reduced under image intensifier control, prior to any incision being made.

A lateral incision is made down to the upper femur. Guide wires are passed up the neck of the femur under image intensifier control and the drill for the screws passed over the guide wires. Two or three screws are inserted up the neck and into the femoral head.

Codes
GA/LA	GA or spinal
Blood	2 units
Antibiotics	Yes
Time	1 hour

Drains	Yes
Plaster	0
Postoperative radiograph	AP pelvis and lateral hip
DVT prophylaxis	Yes
Stay	10–14 days
Follow-up	6 weeks, X-ray on arrival

Operative requirements
- Orthopaedic table.
- Image intensifier and radiographer.

Postoperative care

Management

Remove the drain after 24 hours.

The patient is mobilized fully weight-bearing after the drain has been removed.

Consider the social circumstances of the patient early and refer to the social workers or geriatricians if appropriate.

Complications
- Deep vein thrombosis.
- Pneumonia.
- Urinary tract infection.
- Congestive cardiac failure.
- Failure of fixation.
- Non-union.
- Avascular necrosis of femoral head in 25%.

Operation: hemiarthroplasty for subcapital fracture of the neck of the femur

The hip is approached through an antero-lateral or modified lateral approach. The fractured head is removed and replaced with a prosthesis. The most common types of prostheses used are the Austin-Moore hemiarthroplasty, which is used without cement, and the Thompson's hemiarthroplasty, which is used with cement. Some designs are known as bipolar. These have a small head articulating within a large shell. The aim of these designs is to reduce articulation at the true acetabulum and therefore reduce acetabular wear.

Codes

GA/LA	GA
Blood	2 units
Antibiotics	Yes
Time	1 hour
Drains	Yes
Plaster	0
Postoperative radiograph	AP pelvis and lateral hip
DVT prophylaxis	Yes
Stay	10–14 days
Follow-up	Optional

Postoperative care

Management
Check haemoglobin on postoperative day 2.

Remove the drain after 24–36 hours.

Mobilize the patient after the drain has been removed, according to the surgical approach. The antero-lateral or lateral approaches allow the patient to sit up immediately, as they are stable with the hip flexed.

Cover urinary catheterization with an appropriate antibiotic.

Consider the patient's social circumstances early and if a problem is anticipated, refer to the social workers or geriatrician.

Complications
- Deep vein thrombosis, pneumonia, urinary tract infection, congestive cardiac failure, etc.
- Acetabular wear requiring later revision to a total hip replacement.
- Dislocation.
- Fracture of the femur at or below the tip of the prosthesis.
- Pain on walking.

CHAPTER 63

Fracture of the femoral shaft in a child

Making the diagnosis

The history

The diagnosis is usually obvious. It is important to know the mechanism of injury. If the child has been involved in a road traffic accident there might be other significant injuries. You must look for these. It is all too easy to concentrate on the obvious injury. If the child has suffered a direct blow to the leg, then other trauma is unlikely.

In a toddler, it is always possible that the fracture is the result of a non-accidental injury. Bear this in mind, but do not dwell on the subject.

On examination

Try to establish the diagnosis as quickly and painlessly as possible. Do not try to elicit crepitus at the fracture!

Check that the child has normal neurovascular status distal to the fracture. This is vital in order to exclude a sciatic nerve injury.

Radiographs

Ensure that you have views of both the hip above and the knee below the fracture. Look to see if there is a concomitant hip dislocation or slipped upper femoral epiphysis.

Preoperative management

Common associated injuries
- Multiple injuries.
- Hip dislocation.
- Knee ligament injury.
- Visceral injury.

Preparation for surgery

Make the child comfortable as soon as possible. If the child does not have a head injury, give a single dose of intravenous morphine (0.125 mg/kg estimated body weight). Then insert a femoral nerve block using 0.5% bupivacaine hydrochloride (Marcain) in a dose 1.5 mg/kg estimated body weight. This will allow you to apply skin traction relatively painlessly.

Treatment

For a child who weighs less than 14 kg (30 lb), the definitive management is gallows traction. This set up has the child on his back, with both legs held vertically in skin traction. Enough weight is used to just lift the child's buttocks off the bed. The bandages must be removed daily to check on the condition of the skin, but the adhesive tape of the skin traction should not be disturbed. Once the fracture is 'sticky' and non-tender, a hip spica can be applied.

For a child who weighs more than 14 kg (30 lb), either longitudinal skin traction is used or '90/90' traction via a femoral traction pin. The child has their hip and the knee at 90°

Skin traction can be used in conjunction with a Thomas' splint. Determine the correct splint size by measuring the circumference of the thigh and the leg length of the uninjured side. Then fix on a Pearson knee flexion piece. The splint has to be set up for the appropriate side and it is usually up to the house officer to get the necessary bits and pieces. Use of the Thomas' splint also requires the house officer to check the splint daily and ensure that any pressure pads are correct in their pressure and location.

An alternative is Hamilton Russell traction, which combines below-knee skin traction with a sling placed under the knee. Due to the mechanics of the pulleys, 3 kg (7 lb) weight exerts 6 kg (12 lb) of traction on the leg.

Older children near to closure of their epiphyses, may need skeletal traction via a tibial traction pin and a Thomas' splint. The traction pin is placed lower in the tibia than in an adult, to avoid damaging the tibial apophysis. If necessary the insertion site can be checked with the image intensifier.

The position of the fracture must be checked with weekly radiographs for the first month and then monthly until the fracture is united.

Operation: insertion of tibial traction pin in a child

A Denham pin is inserted through the tibia below the level of the tibial apophysis under a general anaesthetic.

Codes

GA/LA	GA
Blood	Group and save
Antibiotics	Only if the fracture is an open fracture
Time	0.5 hour
Drains	0
Plaster	0
Postoperative radiograph	AP and lateral femur in traction
Stay	1 week per year of age, max. 12 weeks
Follow-up	1 month, X-ray on arrival

Operative requirements

The bed should be ready in theatre with all the traction set-up *before* the child is anaesthetized. This will enable the child to be placed in traction while still anaesthetized. It is up to the doctor to check that everything is correct. Never rely on anyone else.

Image intensifier.

Postoperative care

Management

Start with 4.5 kilograms (10 lb) of traction. Order a check radiograph and adjust the traction accordingly. An overlap of 1.25 mm (0.5 inches) at the fracture is ideal, as the rate of growth of the femur increases following a fracture. If the fracture is brought out to length, the femur may end up longer than the uninjured femur.

The pin sites should be wrapped and left undisturbed so long as they are comfortable.

Complications

- Pin track infection.
- Angular or rotational malunion.
- Leg-length discrepancy.

CHAPTER 64

Fracture of the femoral shaft in an adult

The condition

This is a common fracture. It requires considerable force to break a normal femur. The fracture may be found in a patient with multiple injuries.

Making the diagnosis

On examination

Try to establish the diagnosis as quickly and painlessly as possible. Do not try to elicit crepitus at the fracture!

Check that the neurovascular status is intact distal to the fracture. Feel the pedal pulses, check sensation in the lower leg and foot and ask the patient to move their toes. This is vital to exclude a sciatic nerve or femoral artery injury.

As far as is possible, examine the knee, for bony or ligament injury. The force that fractured the femur may have passed via the knee and injured the latter in the process. If the femur has fractured as a result of the patient's knee hitting the dashboard, you may find that there is either a cruciate ligament rupture or a posterior hip dislocation.

Radiographs

Ensure that the radiographs include views of both the hip above and the knee below the fracture. Look to see if there is a concomitant hip dislocation or fracture of the femoral neck. Look at the lateral view of the knee. Has the tibia fallen back, suggesting a posterior cruciate injury?

Preoperative management

Common associated injuries

- Subcapital femoral neck fracture, hip dislocation or knee ligament injury.
- Sciatic nerve injury.
- Visceral injury.
- Cervical spine injury.

Preparation for surgery

Make sure that there is good venous access – two size 14 cannulae – since closed femoral fractures can lose 4 units of blood into the thigh. In addition there may be an unrecognized injury that is associated with further blood loss.

Treatment

If the patient is not having their fracture stabilized within 6 hours, the leg should be immobilized with skeletal traction via a tibial traction pin.

A femoral fracture may be treated conservatively with skeletal traction (for 3 months). Definitive management for closed fractures is usually internal fixation with an intramedullary nail.

For an open fracture the choice is between an external fixator and an intramedullary nail that is inserted without reaming. The decision depends partly on the size of the wound (see Chapter 3) and partly on the surgeon's preference.

For young adults, we usually remove intramedullary nails 18 months following insertion. This is in case the patient injures the femur again and bends the nail, making it difficult or impossible to remove!

Operation: insertion of tibial traction pin in an adult

The pin is passed through the tibia 2.5 cm (1 inch) inferior and 2.5 cm (1 inch) posterior to the tibial tuberosity, entering on the lateral side. Anaesthetize the entry and exit sites with lignocaine. Use a hand drill to make the track through the tibia with a drill bit that is a little smaller than the Steinmann/Denham pin to be inserted. This will save on your sweat and the patient's pain.

Codes

GA/LA	LA
Blood	4 units
Antibiotics	Only if the fracture is open
Time	30 minutes
Drains	0
Plaster	0
Postoperative radiograph	AP and lateral femur only if traction is definitive management

Operative requirements

A femoral nerve block should be inserted to reduce the pain from the fracture. Much of the discomfort associated with the pin's insertion is due to movement at the fracture site as the pin is pushed through the tibia.

If the pin is to be inserted in casualty, you need to borrow the Steinmann/Denham pin set, a hand drill and some drill bits from theatres. In addition, you need a suture pack, sterile drapes, local anaesthetic, skin prep. and sterile gloves.

Two people are required, one to actually insert the pin, and the other to hold the leg firmly and give counter pressure.

Postoperative care

Management

Skeletal traction is used to keep the patient comfortable until definitive surgery is performed. The traction is set up as the surgeon chooses. 4.5–7 kg/ (10–15/lb) of traction is usually adequate. Traction can be simply straight to a pulley at the end of the bed or the leg may be elevated on a Thomas' splint.

Complication

Pin tract infection.

Operation: intramedullary nail for fractured shaft of femur

In the past a K (Küntscher) nail was used. Nowadays, intramedullary nails can be 'locked' with cross screws (AO nail, G-K or Grosse-Kempf nail, Russell Taylor nail). Locking the nail prevents the bone rotating around the nail and if the fracture is comminuted, prevents the fracture shortening. The nail can be locked proximally, or distally, or both. The choice as to whether to insert locking screws proximally, distally or both depends on the level of the fracture in relation to the isthmus and the configuration of the fracture. The isthmus is the narrow midportion of the femoral shaft.

If the fracture is proximal to the isthmus the nail will only have a good grip in the distal fragment. Therefore, we insert a cross screw in the proximal end of the nail. The nail is then said to be 'locked proximally'.

When the fracture is distal to the isthmus, the nail will only have a good grip in the proximal fragment. We then lock the nail distally.

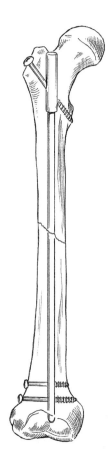

If the fracture is at the isthmus or is comminuted, the nail is locked at both ends to prevent shortening or rotation.

The nail is usually inserted 'closed'. That is to say that the fracture itself is not opened and the procedure is monitored with the image intensifier. We place the patient on the traction table. We apply traction via a femoral traction pin. We usually reduce the fracture before making the incision. We make an incision in the buttock down to the tip of the greater trochanter. We pass a guide wire down the medullary cavity and across the fracture. Reamers are passed over the guide wire to enlarge the medullary cavity. The nail is then passed over the guide wire. To lock the nail, we pass screws across the nail and bone, one proximally and/or two distally.

The nail can be inserted without using a reamer to enlarge the medullary canal. These are known as 'unreamed' nails. They are mainly used for open fractures to reduce the risk of infection. If the fracture is through the subtrochanteric region, the proximal locking screws have to go up the neck into the femoral head. The original nail designed for sub-trochanteric fractures was the *Richards Reconstruction Nail*. As a result any nail that has screws passing up the neck is referred to as a 'recon' nail.

Codes

GA/LA	GA
Blood	3 units
Antibiotics	Yes
Time	1.5 hours
Drains	Yes
Plaster	0
DVT prophylaxis	Yes
Postoperative radiograph	AP and lateral (whole) femur
Stay	10 days
Follow-up	6 weeks
Off work	6 weeks

Operative requirements

- Fracture table.
- Image intensifier and radiographer.
- A femoral traction pin, if not already in skeletal traction.
- Inform theatres as to exactly what type of nail is required.

Postoperative care

Management

Check the haemoglobin on the second postoperative day.

The patient is encouraged to move their hip, knee and ankle immediately.

If the fracture fixation is stable, the patient is allowed to mobilize fully weight-bearing. If unstable, the patient can be mobilized non weight-bearing between crutches.

If the nail is locked at both ends, the patient may need re-admission after 6 weeks, for removal of the screws from one end or the other (often referred to as dynamization). This allows the fracture ends to compress as the patient walks. This encourages fracture healing.

Complications

- Making a simple fracture complex!
- Rotational malalignment.
- Fat embolism.
- Infection.
- Compartment syndrome of the thigh (rare).
- Deep vein thrombosis.
- Loss of position; either shortening or rotational.
- Non-union.

Operation: removal of intramedullary femoral nail

The original incision in the buttock is reopened. The first manoeuvre is to remove any locking screws. Then we have to find the end of the nail. This can be quite difficult if the nail was hammered well down and bone has grown over the entry site. Then the extraction device has to be engaged in the nail and, lastly, the nail must be hammered out. A nail may be so well embedded as to make removal impossible. Removal of a nail often takes longer than its insertion.

Investigations

Make sure that there are recent radiographs of the femur which show union of the fracture and include the upper end of the intramedullary nail.

Codes

GA/LA	GA
Blood	Group and save
Antibiotics	Optional
Time	1 hour
Drains	Yes
Plaster	0
Postoperative radiograph	AP and lateral femur
Stay	Day case or overnight stay
Follow-up	10 days
Off work	2 weeks

Operative requirements

The surgeon must have the correct instruments for extraction of the nail. Therefore the theatre staff must know exactly what kind of nail is to be removed – Küntscher, Grosse-Kempf, AO, Russell Taylor, etc. – and if there are locking screws. If you are in doubt as to the type of nail, look at the old operation note.

Postoperative care

Management

The patient can be mobilized immediately, fully weight-bearing.

Complications

- Fracture not truly united.
- Refracture during nail removal.
- Refracture postoperatively.
- Inability to remove the nail.

CHAPTER 65

Pathological fracture of the femur

The condition

Metastases in the bone are common and are often found in the femur. They typically occur in the subtrochanteric region. The patient may present with pain alone or with a fracture.

Tumours that commonly metastasize to bone are bronchus, breast, prostate, thyroid, kidney and myeloma. Primary bone tumours are much less common.

Making the diagnosis

The history
The patient may have had pain in the hip or thigh for some time prior to the fracture. A pathological fracture is often the first presentation of the malignancy. If this is the case, a thorough history must be taken to try to establish the site of the primary. Also ask the patient if they have any other pains, as these may be due to other bony secondaries.

On examination
Perform a complete and thorough examination to see if there is an obvious primary tumour. This includes a breast examination for women, and a rectal examination for men.

Radiographs
Obtain radiographs of the whole femur to see if there is another lesion in the femur that is not visible on the initial radiographs. If an intramedullary nail is inserted with its tip at the level of an unrecognized lesion, the femur may fracture at the level of the tip of the nail. If a second deposit is found, the nail can then be inserted beyond the lesion.

Investigations

The best screening investigations after a full history and examination are:

- Full blood count.
- Erythrocyte sedimentation rate.
- Urea and electrolytes.
- Liver function tests.
- Acid phosphatase.
- Calcium and alkaline phosphatase.
- Thyroid function tests.
- Serum immunoelectrophoresis.
- Chest radiograph.
- Bone scan.

Preoperative management

Preparation for surgery

In the elderly, skin traction – 2.25 kg (5 lb).

In the young and the middle-aged, skeletal traction via a tibial traction pin.

Always measure the serum calcium preoperatively as hypercalcaemia is common.

Treatment

Indications for surgery

Pathological fractures must be fixed unless the patient is moribund. Fixation may at least provide relief of pain and allow the patient to be nursed in bed without traction. At best, it allows immediate mobilization and thus a better quality of life.

Operation: internal fixation of pathological fractured shaft of femur

The implant used depends on the fracture, the surgeon and the devices available. Choices of implant include a variety of intramedullary nails that all have some sort of locking device. These include the Reconstruction nail and AO nail. Alternatively, if the fracture looks as though it may be stable once fixed, a long nail-plate may suffice. The operative technique is the same as for non-pathological fractures, except that the fracture is exposed so that a specimen of bone can be taken for histology.

Codes

GA/LA	GA
Blood	4 units
Antibiotics	Yes
Time	1.5 hours
Drains	Yes
Plaster	0
DVT prophylaxis	Yes
Postoperative radiograph	AP and lateral femur
Stay	2 weeks
Follow-up	6 weeks

Operative requirements
- Orthopaedic traction table.
- Image intensifier and radiographer.

Postoperative care

Management

Mobilize the patient as soon as their pain allows. Refer the patient to an oncologist if the tumour is sensitive to radiotherapy. It is usually best to wait for the skin to heal before starting radiotherapy.

Monitor the serum calcium, especially if the patient becomes confused or drowsy.

Complications

Beware multiple secondaries. Pain at the site of a known secondary often implies an impending fracture. This may benefit from prophylactic fixation.

Beware hypercalcaemia that can cause acute confusion and may be difficult to treat.

CHAPTER

66

Supracondylar fracture of the femur

The condition

This is not a common fracture. It requires considerable force to break a normal femur. The fracture may be found in a patient with multiple injuries. The fracture also occurs in elderly patients as the result of low energy trauma, such as a fall.

Making the diagnosis

On examination

The knee is usually very swollen and the leg may lie in valgus or varus. There may be a considerable haemarthrosis. Check the neuro-vascular integrity of the lower limb. If there is numbness in the leg or toes, this may be due to direct trauma to either the sciatic nerve, or the lateral popliteal nerve. Note the presence and location of any wounds or fracture blisters.

Radiographs

Order an AP and lateral views of the whole femur.
The key to decision making is whether or not the fracture extends into the knee joint.

Preoperative management

Preparation for surgery

If surgery is unlikely to be performed within a few hours of admission the limb should be immobilized on a Thomas splint with 2.25 kg (5 lb) of skin traction. If surgery is likely to be delayed more than 24 hours, it is best to place a tibial traction pin in the shaft of the tibia and place the limb on skeletal traction on a Braun frame. 4.5 kg (10 lb) of traction should be adequate. This will make the patient much more comfortable and prevent the fracture shortening.

Treatment

The majority of supracondylar fractures are treated operatively. If the fracture extends into the knee joint, the articular surface has to be reduced anatomically.

There are two methods of fixing these fractures. One is to apply a plate and screws to the outside of the femur. The device generally used is the AO *Dynamic Condylar Screw* (DCS).

The alternative is to insert an intramedullary nail. If the fracture does not involve the knee and is not too far distal, a locking nail can be inserted antegrade – from above. The more common alternative is to insert the nail up from below. The supracondylar nail can be used for intra-articular fractures.

Indications for surgery
A displaced fracture of the distal femur.

Contra-indications to surgery
Soft tissue injury over the line of the incision.
An immobile patient who did not walk prior to fracturing their femur.
An unreconstructable fracture.

Operation: open reduction and internal fixation supracondylar fracture using a dynamic condylar screw (DCS)

We make a lateral incision that starts mid thigh and extends to just below the knee. If the fracture goes into the knee, we open the knee and reduce the articular surface anatomically. We insert a large screw parallel to the joint under image intensifier control. The screw is similar to the lag screw of a DHS. We slide the barrel of the plate onto the screw and then fix the plate to the shaft of the femur.

Codes

GA/LA	GA
Blood	2 units
Antibiotics	Yes
Time	1–2 hours
Drains	Yes
Plaster	0

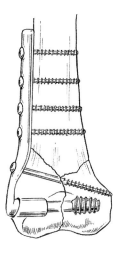

Postoperative radiograph	AP and lateral femur
DVT prophylaxis	Yes
Stay	2 weeks
Follow-up	6 weeks
Off work	3 months

Operative requirements

- High thigh tourniquet.
- AO DCS set.

Operation: internal fixation of supracondylar fracture using a supracondylar nail

If the fracture does not extend into the knee joint, the fracture is reduced closed. In other words the fracture itself is not exposed. We reduce the fracture indirectly, checking the position with the image intensifier. We make a 3 cm incision through the patellar tendon. We make a hole just above the intercondylar notch and insert the nail from distal to proximal. The nail is locked with cross screws at both ends.

If the fracture does go into the knee joint we make a straight midline incision. We reduce the fracture under direct vision and hold the fracture with screws. We then make a hole just above the intercondylar notch and insert the nail from distal to proximal. The nail is locked with cross screws at both ends.

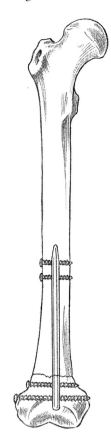

Codes

GA/LA	GA
Blood	2 units
Antibiotics	Yes
Time	1 hour
Drains	No
Plaster	0
Postoperative radiograph	AP and lateral femur
DVT prophylaxis	Yes
Stay	2 weeks
Follow-up	6 weeks
Off work	3 months

Operative requirements
- High thigh tourniquet.
- Image intensifier and radiographer.
- Supracondylar nail set.

Postoperative care

Management

Remove the drains after 24 hours.

If the surgeon is happy with the fixation, the patient may start mobilizing the knee immediately on the CPM machine. Once the sutures are out and the patient has a good range of movement, the leg is protected with a hinged cast brace.

Patients usually remain non weight-bearing for a minimum of 6 weeks.

Complications
- Compartment syndrome.
- Infection.
- Deep vein thrombosis.
- Loss of fixation.
- Restricted range of movement.
- Late osteoarthritis.

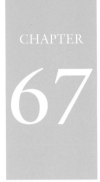

Fracture of the patella

The condition

This fracture usually results from a fall onto a flexed knee.

Making the diagnosis

The patient
It mainly occurs in the middle-aged and elderly.

On examination
There may be a bruise at the site of impact.

If the fracture fragments are displaced, you should be able to feel a gap between them.

There may be some boggy swelling, but there is not normally a large haemarthrosis. If the fracture fragments are displaced, the quadriceps expansion must be torn. Therefore blood disperses and is not kept within the knee joint itself.

See if the patient is able to extend their knee actively. This is best demonstrated by gently flexing the patent's knee a little. Then ask the patient to lift their heel off the bed. Active extension is lost with a displaced fracture of the patella.

Radiographs
AP and lateral views of the knee will show the fracture.

Most fractures are transverse, but some are comminuted. If on the lateral view, the two poles of the patella are widely separated, the quadriceps expansion must be ruptured.

Make sure that what seems like an oblique fracture of the upper part of the patella is not a bipartite patella. This is an ossification centre that remains separate from the rest of the patella and is generally present bilaterally. Therefore order a radiograph of the other knee to see if the uninjured patella is similar in appearance.

Preoperative management

Preparation for surgery
While waiting for surgery, place the leg in a back-slab with the knee extended.

Treatment

A completely undisplaced fracture is treated conservatively, with the leg immobilized in a long leg cylinder for 6 weeks. Radiographs must be taken at 1 and 2 weeks to ensure that the fracture has not displaced.

If the fracture is displaced, continuity of the quadriceps mechanism must be restored. If the patella is in two or three major fragments, it is usually possible to reconstruct the patella.

If it is a very comminuted fracture, the patella may have to be excised.

There may be one large proximal fragment and several small distal fragments. In this case, the small fragments are removed and the patellar tendon is wired to the remaining large proximal patellar fragment.

Indications for surgery
A fractured patella that is displaced.
Inability to perform a straight-leg raise.

Operation: tension band wiring of fractured patella

We make a longitudinal midline incision. The fracture is reduced and then held with two parallel K-wires around which is passed a flexible wire. The ends of the flexible wire are twisted together. It is called 'tension band wiring' because instead of flexion of the knee putting tension on the repair and pulling it apart, the construct converts the force into one that compresses the fracture.

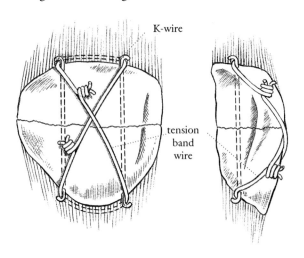

Codes

GA/LA	GA
Blood	0
Antibiotics	Yes
Time	1 hour
Drains	Yes
Plaster	Back-slab
DVT prophylaxis	Yes
Postoperative radiograph	AP and lateral knee
Stay	1 week
Follow-up	6 weeks
Off work	6 weeks

Operative requirements

- K-wiring set.
- High thigh tourniquet.

Postoperative care

Management

The knee is rested in a back-slab for 2 or 3 days. The patient is then mobilized, partially weight bearing between crutches. The back-slab may be used to give extra support. Four or five days after surgery, when the wound is stable and if the fixation is sufficiently solid, active flexion and extension exercises can be started. The continuous passive motion (CPM) machine may then also be used.

Complications

- Inadequate fixation.
- Wound breakdown.
- Late osteoarthritis if the fracture cannot be reduced anatomically.
- Discomfort over the wires, necessitating their removal after the fracture has healed.

CHAPTER 68

Arthritis of the knee

The condition

Osteoarthritis of the knee may be secondary to previous intra-articular trauma, meniscectomy, crystal arthropathy or simple obesity. The knee is commonly affected by rheumatoid arthritis.

Making the diagnosis

The patient
The patient is usually middle- or old-aged. An elderly patient may have problems in other joints as well as medical problems. One has to ensure that giving them a pain-free knee will allow them greater mobility. For example, if the patient has severe angina, a knee replacement may not significantly improve their quality of life. In addition the operation will be hazardous to their health.

The history
Ask about any previous knee problems or operations.

The most significant complaint is pain. Establish the following:

- For how long can the patient walk, before the pain makes them stop?
- Does knee pain wake the patient?
- What analgesics does the patient take and how often?
- Does the knee give way, swell or lock?
- How does the patient go up stairs? Normally, or one stair at a time?

If the patient has rheumatoid arthritis, consider whether problems in other joints will limit his mobility following surgery. Also ascertain whether the knee pain is worse than any hip pain that he may have.

On examination
Watch the patient walk. Note any limp and how a stick is used.

Look at the alignment of the leg. Is there a varus or valgus deformity when the patient is standing?

Look for scars from previous surgery to the knee. The patient may forget to mention an operation if it was many years previously.

Examine the knee to see if any swelling is due to osteophytes or an effusion or both.

Check the integrity of the collateral ligaments. If the medial collateral ligament is intact, a varus knee that is due to medial joint collapse can usually be brought straight and then an endpoint is felt. This is different to a knee that can be brought into varus due to laxity of the lateral collateral ligament.

Examine the range of flexion and extension, and in particular the presence of a flexion contracture and/or the inability to flex the knee beyond 90°.

Do not omit to examine the movements of the hips and the neurological and vascular status of both limbs.

Note any signs of venous stasis that imply previous venous problems, especially a deep vein thrombosis.

If the patient has rheumatoid arthritis, examine all the major joints, especially the neck and temporomandibular joint.

Radiographs

Obtain AP and lateral radiographs of the knees. The AP should be a standing film of both legs. This allows the surgeon to see the true varus/valgus deformity. Request an AP pelvis to ensure that the knee pain is not referred from an arthritic hip joint.

If the patient has rheumatoid arthritis, obtain views of the cervical spine.

Preoperative management

Investigations

Always obtain a midstream urine for microscopy, culture and sensitivity in a patient undergoing prosthetic replacement.

Treatment

The initial treatment for all arthritic joints is medical. This includes analgesics and anti-inflammatory drugs, as well as physiotherapy. The use of a walking stick and a non-steroidal anti-inflammatory drug may be enough to relieve the pain in many patients.

Indications for surgery

The primary aim of any surgery for arthritis is to relieve pain. Although there may be improved movement or stability, these are secondary benefits and not the reason for performing surgery.

A high tibial osteotomy may be performed for medial compartment osteoarthritis in the knee of a relatively young person (less than 60 years). The aim of the osteotomy is to correct deformity and shift some of the load away from the diseased part of the joint.

Even a perfectly performed osteotomy cannot guarantee complete resolution of symptoms. Although there is usually an improvement in the patient that can last for years, it will not last for ever. Most patients will need a total knee replacement in the future.

Degeneration that is confined to either the medial or the lateral compartment may be suitable for a unicondylar knee arthroplasty.

Joint destruction throughout the knee, accompanied by severe pain, is treated with a total knee replacement.

If a knee replacement becomes infected or loose, it is revised if at all possible. However, this is not always possible and the knee may have to be fused.

Contra-indications to surgery

Minimal symptoms, however severe the radiographic changes.

Severe flexion contracture.

Ischaemic heart disease or peripheral vascular disease that would obscure the benefits of knee replacement; i.e. if angina or claudication are so severe that the patient will not be able to walk very far following surgery, the risks may outweigh the benefits.

Urinary tract infection.

Prostatism that may result in postoperative urinary retention and the need for a prostatectomy. It is better to have the urological investigations and surgery before a knee replacement.

Operation: high tibial osteotomy

Using either a midline or transverse incision, an osteotomy is made in the upper tibia about 2.5 cm (1 inch) below the joint. For medial compartment disease, a wedge of bone is removed that is laterally based. The gap is closed and the osteotomy is held with one or two staples. This is a very stable arrangement and the patient's knee can be mobilized out of plaster postoperatively. A CPM machine may be used initially after surgery. If a dome-shaped cut is made to realign the tibia, the patient stays in plaster while the osteotomy unites.

Codes

GA/LA	GA
Blood	2 units
Antibiotics	Yes
Time	1.5 hours
Drains	Yes
Plaster	Yes
DVT prophylaxis	Yes
Postoperative radiograph	AP and lateral upper tibia
Stay	10 days
Follow-up	6 weeks
Off work	3 months

Operative requirements

A high thigh tourniquet.

If the osteotomy is to be held with a staple, this should be specified on the operating list.

Postoperative care

Management

Measure the haemoglobin on the second postoperative day.

Mobilization depends on the exact method of fixation and the stability of the osteotomy. The surgeon should state the regimen in his postoperative instructions.

Complications

- Inadequate correction.
- Loss of fixation and position.
- Infection.
- Deep vein thrombosis.
- Persistent pain.

Operation: total knee replacement

We make an vertical midline skin incision. We divide the medial capsule medially and reflect the patella laterally. Each make or design of knee replacement has specific cutting guides for preparing the bone. The surfaces of the femoral condyles, the tibial plateau and the patella are trimmed using a powered saw and the cutting guides. The modern prostheses are essentially surface replacements and we remove the minimum amount of bone necessary to obtain a good fit. The anterior cruciate is usually 'sacrificed'. The posterior cruciate ligament may or may not be retained, depending on the design of the knee replacement. The collateral ligaments are preserved as they are essential to the stability of these 'unconstrained' designs. The components articulate with each other, but are not linked. Whether or not the surface of the patella is replaced varies from surgeon to surgeon.

The components of the knee replacement are usually cemented in place using bone cement. Some prostheses are designed to be inserted without cement. Uncemented knee arthroplasty is preferable in the younger patient who is more likely to need revision surgery than an older patient.

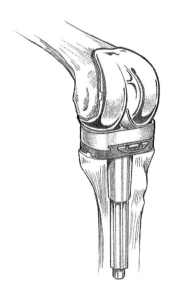

Codes

GA/LA	GA
Blood	3 units
Antibiotics	Yes
Time	1.5 hours
Drains	Yes
Plaster	0
DVT prophylaxis	Yes
Postoperative radiograph	AP and lateral knee
Stay	10 days
Follow-up	6 weeks
Off work	3 months

Operative requirement
The tourniquet has to be as high as possible on the thigh.

Postoperative care

Management
Unless the tourniquet was deflated prior to closure, a knee replacement can drain up to 500 ml in the first few postoperative hours, so do not panic.

Check the foot pulses and sensation immediately after surgery. Document your findings in the notes.

Remove the drains after 24 hours.

Check the haemoglobin on postoperative day 2.

The patient is encouraged to mobilize his knee immediately after the operation. The physiotherapy may be supplemented with a CPM machine.

The patient is allowed to begin walking, fully weight-bearing as soon as they are comfortable enough. This is usually after 2 days. If they do not have good quadriceps control and cannot do a straight-leg raise they may need a brace on their knee.

Complications
- Neuro-vascular injury.
- Wound infection.
- Deep vein thrombosis.
- Deep infection of the prosthesis.
- Late loosening.

Operation: revision of total knee replacement

Revision of a total knee replacement is considerably more difficult and hazardous than the primary operation.

If the original replacement is loose, there may be considerable bony erosion. This can make implanting the revision prosthesis very difficult. All the original cement has to be removed, but this is not as difficult as in a revision hip replacement. Special revision prostheses are used which are designed to compensate for the loss of bone. The prostheses usually have longer stems to aid fixation of both the femoral and the tibial components.

If the original prosthesis is being removed for infection, bone loss is usually less of a problem. Cement removal however, must be meticulous. The infected components are removed, but the new prosthesis is not inserted immediately. Instead, either beads or a spacer of antibiotic-impregnated cement are left in the wound. The patient is given an appropriate systemic antibiotic for 6 weeks. The knee is then reopened and the new components inserted.

Codes

GA/LA	GA
Blood	4 units
Antibiotics	Yes
Time	2 hours
Drains	Yes
Plaster	0
DVT prophylaxis	Yes
Postoperative radiograph	AP and lateral knee
Stay	3 weeks
Follow-up	6 weeks
Off work	3 months

Operative requirement
High thigh tourniquet.

Postoperative care

Management
Remove the drains after 24 hours (NB they always drain a lot in the first few hours unless the tourniquet was deflated prior to closure).

270

Check the haemoglobin on postoperative day 2.

Many surgeons rest the knee extended in a back-slab, until the wound is stable. The knee is then mobilized with or without the CPM machine.

The patient is allowed to begin walking fully weight-bearing, when he has good quadriceps control and is able to straight-leg raise.

Complications

- Intraoperative fracture of femur or tibia.
- Inability to insert new prosthesis.
- Neuro-vascular injury.
- Wound infection.
- Deep infection of the prosthesis.
- Deep vein thrombosis.
- Late loosening.

Operation: arthrodesis of the knee

The knee is usually fused following failure of a total knee arthroplasty. The prosthesis is removed and the bone surfaces are cleaned of all debris and cement. If necessary, iliac crest bone graft is inserted into the gap between femur and tibia to encourage the bones to fuse. The knee is then held by one of two alternative methods. Either a stout intramedullary nail is passed from the femur into the tibia, or an external fixator is applied.

Codes

GA/LA	GA
Blood	2 units
Antibiotics	Yes
Time	1 hour
Drains	Yes
Plaster	Only with external fixator
DVT prophylaxis	Yes
Postoperative radiographer	AP and lateral knee radiograph if external clamp used; AP and lateral femur and tibia if intramedullary nail used
Stay	2–3 weeks
Follow-up	6 weeks
Off work	3 months

Operative requirements

If an intramedullary nail is used it must be long enough! Nails are available up to 700 mm in length but it is worth checking that a long nail is available.

If an external fixator is to be used, ensure that a complete set is available.

Postoperative care

Management

If an external fixator is used, an above-knee plaster may be needed for extra stability. Initially the patient must remain non weight-bearing. The transverse pins are removed after 6 weeks and a plaster cylinder is applied in which the patient can weight bear. The plaster stays on for a further 6 weeks.

If an intramedullary nail is used, the patient can fully weight bear immediately.

Complications

- Wound infection.
- Failure to fuse.
- Fracture of the tibia or femur at the tip of the nail.

69 Patello-femoral arthritis

The condition

Arthritis that mainly affects the patello-femoral joint is unusual in isolation, but can follow chondromalacia patellae or trauma. It is more common to have severe patello-femoral arthritis combined with minimal degenerative change in the rest of the knee.

Making the diagnosis

The history
The patient complains of pain that is maximal behind the patella and worse on walking up and down stairs.

On examination
The main finding of note, apart from the scars of previous operations, is the crepitus that you can feel when you move the patella from side to side with a little downwards pressure. This is usually accompanied by pain.

Radiographs
Lateral and skyline views of the knee show a loss of joint space between the patella and the femur, and osteophytes on the patella.

Treatment

Indications for surgery
Surgery is only warranted for severe degeneration of the articular surface of the patello-femoral joint that is accompanied by severe pain. If the degenerative change is truly confined to the patello-femoral joint, then the only option at present is to excise the patella.

Operation: excision of the patella

We make either a transverse or a longitudinal midline skin incision. We shell out the patella carefully, taking care to preserve the vertical fibres of the quadriceps. The continuity of the quadriceps expansion is thus maintained.

Codes

GA/LA	GA
Blood	Group and save
Antibiotics	Yes
Time	1 hour
Drains	Yes
Plaster	Yes, cylinder
Postoperative radiograph	0
Stay	2 weeks
Follow-up	6 weeks
Off work	3 months

Operative requirement
High thigh tourniquet.

Postoperative care

Management
Static quadriceps exercises are started immediately after surgery.

The patient can be placed on a CPM machine immediately.

The patient is allowed to walk when they are able to perform a straight-leg raise, their pain has settled and the range of motion of their knee is satisfactory.

Complications
- Extension lag – the patient raises the leg in slight flexion when trying to raise the leg straight.
- Loss of full flexion.

70 Torn meniscus in the knee

The condition

This is a common injury.

Patients are often confused when doctors talk about cartilage. In lay terms, patients refer to having a torn 'cartilage'. The patient understands that a cartilage is a structure within a joint that can be torn. It is worth explaining to the patient that when doctors talk about cartilage that they are referring to the lining of the joint that covers the bone. This is different from the two menisci that are structures within the joint. This helps avoid confusion when a patient is told that the cartilage of the joint is intact but that their torn meniscus has been removed.

The medial meniscus is more commonly injured than the lateral.

There are different patterns of meniscal tears. A bucket handle tear is tear parallel to the free edge of the meniscus with the ends remaining intact. This 'bucket handle' can flip in and out of the middle of the joint and give rise to locking. With a horizontal cleavage tear, the plane of the tear is parallel to the flat surface of the meniscus. It does not need to be removed. A parrot beak tear is a split in either the anterior or posterior horn of the meniscus.

Making the diagnosis

The patient
Children very rarely injure their menisci.

In young active adults, most symptomatic tears occur after a significant injury.

Less force is required to tear the meniscus in the older patient.

The history

In the young active adult, the meniscus is torn by a twisting injury to the flexed, weight-bearing knee. This may occur during games such as football, when the patient has all their weight on one leg with the knee bent and is twisting at the same time. Usually a sharp pain is felt in the knee, but it does not stop them from finishing their game. The knee swells over several hours or overnight, although not dramatically. If the patient is not treated and returns to sports, he may complain of pain over the medial or lateral joint line after activity.

The knee may lock. True locking occurs if the knee cannot be fully extended due to a mechanical block, but can be flexed almost fully. Without treatment, a knee may remain locked for days and then spontaneously unlock, often while the patient is asleep. You must distinguish this from what patients describe as locking. This is when pain in the knee prevents them from flexing their extended knee.

A more severe injury, such as a skiing accident, may result in 'the unhappy triad' – torn medial meniscus, torn anterior cruciate ligament and ruptured medial collateral ligament (see Chapter 71).

On examination

A full examination of the acutely injured knee is not usually possible since this causes too much discomfort. If the knee is not locked and there is not a huge effusion (which would otherwise suggest a ruptured anterior cruciate ligament), the knee is best examined after it has been rested for about 10 days.

Look for an effusion and quadriceps wasting.

Examine the range of movement of both knees. Many people normally have a degree of recurvatum. If you lift a patient's heel off the couch, the normal knee usually hyper-extends a few degrees. It is significant if this has been lost on the injured side.

Flex the knee and examine for tenderness along the joint line.

Perform McMurray's test. This is impossible to describe and is best demonstrated!

Check on the integrity of the anterior cruciate ligament by performing an anterior draw with the knee flexed at 90° and a Lachmann's test with the knee flexed 10°.

Examine the collateral ligaments.

Radiographs

Radiographs of the knee should be ordered but are normal if the meniscal tear is the only injury.

Preoperative management

Investigations

Some surgeons like to confirm the clinical diagnosis of a meniscal tear with an MR scan. Their aim is to reduce the number of arthroscopies performed on normal knees.

Common associated injuries

Torn anterior cruciate ligament and/or the medial collateral ligament.

Treatment

If there is a tense haemarthrosis or the knee is truly locked, the knee should be arthroscoped on the next convenient operating list to establish the source of the bleeding or the cause of the locking. A patient with a knee that repeatedly locks or gives way, should undergo an elective arthroscopy.

Indications for surgery

Presumed internal derangement in the knee, e.g. meniscal tear.
Prelude to a further procedure, e.g. unicondylar knee replacement or anterior cruciate ligament reconstruction.

Contra-indications to surgery

Complete resolution of symptoms.

Operation: arthroscopy of the knee

Under a general anaesthetic, the knee is viewed using an arthroscope. This is a fibre-optic telescope that is approximately 5 mm wide and is inserted via a small stab incision. The whole of the inside of the knee joint can be inspected. Special instruments can be introduced into the knee via other small incisions. The arthroscope can be linked to a video camera so that the image is displayed on a television monitor for all to see. The camera allows an assistant to hold the arthroscope, leaving the surgeon free to operate with both hands.

Although one can usually excise a torn meniscus using the arthroscope it is not always possible. The surgeon may have to make a 2.5 cm (1 inch) incision to perform an open meniscectomy. Therefore, if the arthroscopy is being performed for a probable torn meniscus, you must consent the patient for an arthroscopic partial meniscectomy, *and possible open meniscectomy*. Patients who have undergone an open procedure have a longer recovery period, both as an inpatient and as an outpatient.

Arthroscopy of the acutely injured knee is not easy. Extra care has to be taken if the collateral ligament is disrupted since the capsule will also be torn. This capsular tear allows the irrigation fluid to run out of the knee into the calf and may result in a compartment syndrome.

Codes

GA/LA	GA
Blood	0
Antibiotics	0
Time	45 minutes
Drains	0
Plaster	0
Postoperative radiograph	0
Stay	Day case
Follow-up	1 week
Off work	Few days

Operative requirement
High thigh tourniquet.

Postoperative care

Management
If no procedure other than looking inside the knee is performed, the patient can go home the same or next day with crutches.

If an arthroscopic procedure (e.g. partial meniscectomy) is performed, this can still can be done as a day-case. However, the length of the procedure and anaesthetic may necessitate overnight admission.

Sometimes, due to difficulty in removing the meniscus arthroscopically, it is necessary to actually open the knee through a formal arthrotomy. If so, the patient has to remain in hospital until he can straight-leg raise and is able to walk.

Complications
- Missed lesion, leading to persistent symptoms.
- Infection.

CHAPTER 71

Rupture of the anterior cruciate ligament

The condition

Rupture of the anterior cruciate ligament is common. The patient may be seen immediately following the injury. Alternatively the diagnosis may be made when the patient complains of pain and instability weeks or months after the acute episode.

Making the diagnosis

The patient
The patient is usually a young adult who injures his knee while skiing or playing football.

The history
The typical history is of a twisting injury to the knee with immediate pain. There is gross swelling of the knee within half an hour of the injury. This is pathognomonic of either a torn anterior cruciate ligament or an intra-articular fracture. The patient is unable to continue the activity and hobbles off the football field or is carried off the ski slope.

If the patient is seen sometime after the acute episode, he complains of a feeling of instability that is most marked on going down stairs. The knee may swell and ache after sports. Locking is not typical of a ruptured anterior cruciate ligament. Remember, however, that the medial meniscus and the medial collateral ligament may be injured at the same time as the anterior cruciate ligament, as part of 'the unhappy triad'.

On examination
There is usually a haemarthrosis following rupture of the anterior cruciate ligament. This may remain for up to 2 weeks and the severe pain

that accompanies the haemarthrosis prevents a complete examination of the knee.

If you examine the patient's knee after the acutely painful period, you should be able to elicit some or all of the following signs of a ruptured anterior cruciate:

(a) a positive Lachmann's test;

(b) a positive anterior draw sign;

(c) a positive pivot shift.

Always examine the integrity of the collateral ligaments and perform a McMurray's test to examine the menisci.

Radiographs

If the bony origin of the anterior cruciate origin has been avulsed from the tibia, the bony fragment may be visible on radiographs of the knee. On the AP view, the fragment may be seen in the intercondylar notch and on the lateral view, it may lie just above the anterior tibial plateau.

A fluid level may be seen on the lateral view of the knee. This is due to a lipo-haemarthrosis. It is most easily detected if you orientate the radiograph with the knee horizontal. This is how the film was taken and the fluid/fat line will be horizontal.

Common associated injuries

Medial meniscus bucket handle tear.

Rupture of the medial collateral ligament.

Treatment

If a patient has a tense haemarthrosis and is not going directly to theatre, aspirate the joint using a full aseptic no-touch technique. This will provide great relief of pain as well as confirming the presence of blood in the knee.

Indications for surgery

Some surgeons like to take all patients with a haemarthrosis to theatre to wash out the joint, perform an arthroscopy and establish the exact diagnosis.

Reconstruction procedures for complete rupture of the anterior cruciate ligament are indicated in a young adult with severe symptoms. The patient must be prepared for several months of postoperative physiotherapy. The diagnosis of a ruptured anterior cruciate ligament may be confirmed at arthroscopy prior to reconstruction, or an MRI may suffice.

Some surgeons believe that stabilizing the knee may reduce the incidence of later osteoarthritis.

Operation: Jones's reconstruction of the anterior cruciate ligament; Macintosh's antero-lateral stabilization of the knee

In the Jones's reconstruction of the anterior cruciate ligament, the middle third of the patella tendon is removed with bone attached at either end. A hole is drilled through the upper tibia and exits at the point of origin of the anterior cruciate ligament on the tibial plateau. Another hole is drilled starting at the point of the ACL's attachment to the medial side of the lateral femoral condyle and exiting out the lateral side of the shaft of femur. The 'graft' is passed up through the tibial hole, across the knee joint and out the femoral hole. Special screws are used to hold the bone on either end of the tendon graft within the holes in the tibia and femur. The aim is to replicate the path of the deficient ligament.

Codes

GA/LA	GA
Blood	0
Antibiotics	Yes
Time	1.5 hours
Drains	Yes
Plaster	0
Postoperative radiograph	AP and lateral knee
Stay	Overnight
Follow-up	6 weeks
Off work	6 weeks minimum

Operative requirement
High thigh tourniquet.

Postoperative care

Management
Some surgeons prefer that the patient wears a hinged knee brace postoperatively. The surgeon will state what range of flexion he will allow. The patient may have to wear the brace for 6 weeks.

The patient is discharged from hospital once they are safe walking with crutches.

Complications
- Neurovascular injury.
- Compartment syndrome.
- Lax reconstruction leading to persistent symptoms.
- Permanent loss of full extension.
- Patella fracture.

CHAPTER 72

Chondromalacia patellae

The condition

Chondromalacia literally means soft (articular) cartilage. The cartilage becomes soft, soggy and irregular. This may be due to a single injury to the cartilage. More commonly it is due to faulty tracking of the patella over the femoral condyle during flexion of the knee. This results in excessive pressure on the cartilage. The true nature of the condition is not known. Furthermore, why only the patellar side of the patello-femoral joint is affected is not understood.

Making the diagnosis

The patient
Chondromalacia patella is a frequent problem in teenage girls, but not exclusively so.

The history
The patient complains of a diffuse pain in the front of the knee without having suffered any specific injury. The knee does not truly lock or give way.

On examination
There may be a slight effusion.

With the patient's knee extended, palpate the articular surface of the patella. By pushing the patella medially and then laterally you can examine a large part of the articular surface. There may be a specific area that is tender.

Radiographs
Radiographs of the knee should be ordered. However, they are usually normal.

Treatment

The initial treatment is always conservative. The patient is advised to avoid excessive activity and to take a non-steroidal anti-inflammatory drug. In most cases the pain settles without invasive treatment. It may take more than a year for the pain to settle. If the pain persists, the knee can be arthroscoped to confirm the diagnosis. If an area of cartilage is found to be very abnormal it may be curetted and drilled arthroscopically. This can give relief of pain that may or may not be permanent. In most cases the cartilage is softer than normal but is not dramatically abnormal.

If the cause for the chondromalacia seems to be excess lateral pressure, a lateral release may be performed. This is usually performed 'closed' through a small incision. We cut the lateral capsule including the synovium. The cut can be seen via the arthroscope, but is often judged by feel alone.

Operation: lateral release of the knee

The aim of this procedure is to diminish the pressure on the lateral side of the patella by dividing the lateral capsule.

After an arthroscopy, a pair of scissors is inserted through a small skin incision, with one blade within the knee joint and the other outside the capsule (but under the skin). The scissors are run upwards, thus dividing the lateral capsule.

Codes

GA/LA	GA
Blood	0
Antibiotics	0
Time	15 minutes
Drains	0
Plaster	0
Postoperative radiograph	0
Stay	Day case or overnight stay
Follow-up	2 weeks
Off work	2 weeks

Operative requirements
- High thigh tourniquet.
- Arthroscope.

Postoperative care

Management
A firm wool and crêpe bandage is kept on the knee for at least 48 hours as there is a risk of bleeding from the lateral geniculate vessels. If the knee is kept extended, the lateral structures that have been divided may repair themselves. Therefore, the patient is encouraged to flex the knee immediately.

Complications
- Haemarthrosis.
- Incomplete resolution of symptoms.

73

Cyst of the lateral meniscus

The condition

The cause of cysts of the lateral meniscus is unknown. It has been suggested that they may develop as a sequel to previous trauma. Meniscal cysts are commonly associated with a tear of the lateral meniscus and the clinical features may be those of a meniscal tear. The neck of the cyst usually communicates with the knee joint.

Making the diagnosis

The patient
The patient is a young adult, more commonly male than female.

The history
The main complaint is of a hard lump on the lateral aspect of the knee. The patient may complain of a bony lump. There may be an ache associated with the lump.

On examination
What the patient describes as a 'bony' lump is in fact a swelling on the antero-lateral joint line that is largest and hardest with the knee flexed to 90°. With the leg fully extended the lump may disappear altogether.

Radiographs
Radiographs of the knee should be ordered, but are generally normal.

Treatment

Indication for surgery
A cyst that is painful and persists can be excised surgically.

Operation: excision of a cyst of the lateral meniscus

Opinions vary on how best to remove these cysts. Some surgeons simply excise the cyst down to and into the joint. Some surgeons perform an arthroscopy and decompress the cyst from within.

Most surgeons arthroscope the knee to ensure that there is no associated tear in the lateral meniscus. They then make an incision directly over the cyst and excise it.

Codes

GA/LA	GA
Blood	0
Antibiotics	0
Time	1 hour
Drains	0
Plaster	0
Postoperative radiograph	0
Stay	Day case or overnight
Follow-up	10 days
Off work	2 weeks

Operative requirements

- Thigh tourniquet.
- Arthroscopy equipment.

Postoperative care

Management

The patient mobilizes, fully weight-bearing, when they are able to perform a straight-leg raise.

Complications

- Haemarthrosis from intra-articular bleeding.
- Recurrence of the cyst.

Fracture of the tibial plateau

The condition

In the younger patient, this fracture results from a high energy injury and may be one of multiple injuries. The fracture also occurs in elderly patients as the result of low energy trauma, such as a minor fall.

Making the diagnosis

On examination

The patient's knee is usually very swollen and the leg may lie in valgus or varus. There may be a large haemarthrosis.

Check the neuro-vascular integrity of the lower limb. If the leg or toes are numb, this may be due to direct trauma to a nerve, commonly the lateral popliteal, or due to a developing compartment syndrome.

Note the presence and location of any wounds or fracture blisters.

Radiographs

Order AP and lateral views of the knee.

You may also need oblique views, and/or AP and lateral tomograms to visualize the configuration of the fracture fragments. Alternatively a CT scan, preferably with reconstruction views, will show the configuration of the fracture.

The amount of depression of the articular surface has to be assessed since it is this that may require surgical correction.

Preoperative management

Preparation for surgery

If the patient requires surgery, immobilize the leg in a back-slab.

If massive swelling or fracture blisters prevent surgery being performed within 48 hours, it is best to insert a calcaneal traction pin and apply skeletal traction. 4.5 kg (10 lb) of traction should be adequate.

If the patient is not having immediate surgery and there is a large haemarthrosis, it should be drained using a meticulous aseptic, no-touch technique. This will make the patient much more comfortable.

Treatment

An elderly patient with a minimally displaced fracture should be admitted. The limb is either immobilized in a plaster cylinder or mobilized on the CPM machine. The choice depends on the patient and the availability of the equipment. The patient is mobilized by the physiotherapists after the pain settles.

Indications for surgery
A displaced fracture with depression of the joint surface.

Contra-indications to surgery
Compound injury or soft tissue injury over the line of the incision.

Operation: open reduction and internal fixation of tibial plateau fracture

The aim is restore the articular surface to as near normal as is possible. The fracture fragments are exposed through a midline skin incision. The joint surface is pushed up from below. This creates a bony defect that has to be packed with bone graft. The bone graft is usually taken from an iliac crest. The fragments are held using buttress plates and screws.

Codes

GA/LA	GA
Blood	2 units
Antibiotics	Yes
Time	1–2 hours
Drains	Yes
Plaster	0
Postoperative radiograph	AP and lateral knee
DVT prophylaxis	Yes

Stay	2 weeks
Follow-up	6 weeks
Off work	3 months

Operative requirements
- Obtain consent for and include on the theatre list, the possibility of iliac crest bone graft.
- High thigh tourniquet.
- Standard AO set with buttress plates.

Postoperative care

Management
Remove the drains after 24 hours.

Beware compartment syndrome. If the patient has increasing pain unrelieved by splitting dressings down to the skin, call a more senior person – do not just give stronger analgesics.

If the surgeon is happy with the fixation, mobilize the knee immediately on the CPM machine. Otherwise, the leg is immobilized in a plaster back-slab.

The patient needs to remain non weight-bearing for 12 weeks.

Complications
- Compartment syndrome.
- Infection.
- Deep vein thrombosis.
- Loss of fixation.
- Restricted range of movement.
- Late osteoarthritis.

Fracture of the shaft of the tibia

Making the diagnosis

The patient

This injury can occur at any age. Low velocity trauma produces simple, closed injuries. High energy injuries produce comminuted fractures that may be open and may be accompanied by neurological or vascular damage. Unless the fracture is a result of a direct blow, always consider the patient to have suffered multiple trauma until proved otherwise.

The history

Establish exactly how the injury occurred. If the fracture is open, in what environment did it occur? If it is an open fracture, always inspect the covering garments. The lack of a hole in the trousers at the level of the fracture suggests that contamination is less than if the bone came out through the trousers.

On examination

Look at the limb and at the state of the soft tissue over the fracture. Note and document the presence and location of any fracture blisters. A closed fracture can have such a severe soft tissue injury that the management is as difficult as if it were open.

If there is a wound that has been inspected and dressed, do not re-expose it. Each viewing increases the risk of infection.

Carefully examine the neurological and vascular status of the lower limb.

Examine the range of active and passive movement of the toes. If movement of the toes is accompanied by severe pain, the patient may have a compartment syndrome. If you are worried that the patient may be developing a compartment syndrome, reexamine him an hour after the first examination. Keep reviewing the patient until you are sure he does or does not have a compartment syndrome.

Radiographs

AP and lateral views of the whole tibia are essential. Make sure that both the knee and the ankle can be seen. If the original radiographs are obliques taken in the ambulance service's splint, ask for true AP and lateral views.

Preoperative management

Common associated injuries

- Soft tissue trauma to lower leg.
- Neuro-vascular injury.
- Acute compartment syndrome.

Preparation for surgery

If the leg is grossly deformed, give the patient some analgesia and pull it straight. Do not wait for radiographs to confirm a diagnosis that is clinically obvious.

Place the limb in an above-knee back-slab while awaiting primary treatment.

You may need to insert a calcaneal traction pin. This can be inserted in the accident department under local anaesthetic. Then arrange skeletal traction on a Braun frame with 4.5 kg (10 lb) of traction.

Treatment

An undisplaced fracture can be placed in a plaster cast in the plaster room. The plaster cast should be split. If the patient is comfortable and sensible, he does not need to be admitted. The patient should be observed for 24 hours if you are concerned that he may develop a compartment syndrome or that the patient is unreliable.

Not all displaced fractures need to be reduced. If there is more than 50% overlap of the bone and the overall alignment is satisfactory on both the AP and lateral views, the fracture can be treated conservatively in a plaster cast.

Alternatively, if the fracture is displaced, it may need to be reduced into an acceptable position. Once reduced, the position may be maintained in a plaster cast or internal fixation may be necessary.

Indications for surgery

An open fracture is a surgical emergency. Irrigation and debridement should be performed as soon as possible and certainly within 6 hours following the injury (not arrival in casualty). Once clean, the fracture is immobilized either in plaster, or in skeletal traction, or with an external fixator. The fracture may be fixed with an unreamed intramedullary nail.

Most tibial fractures need some form of intervention, even if only a manipulation. The position is only acceptable if there is no varus/valgus angulation, no rotational deformity and the overlap of the shaft is 50% or more.

If the fracture is unstable or has failed a trial of conservative treatment, it may require internal fixation. This is either by an intramedullary nail or a plate. As a rule, plates and nails are removed 18 months after their insertion.

Operation: manipulation under anaesthesia (MUA) of a fractured shaft of tibia

Some fractures are easily manipulated into an anatomical position. Others can prove impossible to get bony apposition. This may be due to interposition of either tendon or muscle between the fracture ends. Once an acceptable reduction has been achieved, the next manoeuvre is to apply an above-knee plaster without losing the position.

There are several ways to reduce a tibia. You can manipulate the fracture with the lower leg hanging over the end of the operating table. Once the fracture is reduced, you then put on the below-knee part of the plaster before extending the knee to continue the plaster above the knee. Alternatively, you can manipulate the leg with the knee extended and put a block behind the knee, so that the below-knee part of the plaster can be applied. Once the plaster is set, move the block under the calf, and with the knee flexed at 15–20°, continue the plaster to above the knee.

Always split the plaster.

Codes

GA/LA	GA
Blood	0
Antibiotics	0
Time	30 minutes
Drains	0
Plaster	Above knee
DVT prophylaxis	Ask consultant
Postoperative radiograph	AP and lateral tibia
Stay	2 days
Follow-up	1 week, X-ray on arrival
Off work	2–3 months

Operative requirements

- Image intensifier and radiographer.
- Radiolucent operating table.
- An assistant who is skilled at applying plaster.

Postoperative care

Management

Beware compartment syndrome. If the patient has increasing pain unrelieved by splitting the cast *down to the skin*, call a more senior person – do not just give stronger analgesics. A reduced fracture should not hurt much!

Mobilize the patient non weight-bearing with crutches.

Children remain in plaster approximately 1 week for every year of their age, up to a maximum of 12 weeks.

Adults require a minimum of 12 weeks in plaster. The second 6 weeks can be in a below-knee, patella tendon-bearing (Sarmiento) cast, in which they can bear weight.

Complications

- Compartment syndrome.
- Deep vein thrombosis.
- Fat embolism.
- Loss of position.
- Delayed union.

- Malunion.
- Non-union.

Operation: irrigation and debridement of open tibial fracture ± insertion of calcaneal traction pin or application of external fixator

Under a general anaesthetic, the wound edges and all the injured tissue are excised and all dirt removed.

If a motorcyclist comes off at speed and suffers a open tibial fracture, the proximal fragment may dig into the ground forcing dirt high up the medullary canal. One has therefore to deliver the ends of the fracture into the wound and ensure that the medullary canal is free of contamination.

It is best not to close open wounds, however tempting. If the wound has to be extended in order to clean the soft tissue and bone, the surgical extension can be closed. The original wound is left open.

Once the wound is clean, the fracture must be reduced and then immobilized. It may be possible to immobilize a stable fracture with a grade I wound in a long-leg plaster back-slab. All other open tibial fractures are immobilized with traction through a calcaneal traction pin or with an external fixator or with an unreamed intramedullary nail. The aim is to allow unimpeded access to the wound. The decision about which method to use depends on the wound, the surgeon and the apparatus available:

A calcaneal traction pin is generally inserted if the wound looks as though it may be possible for it to be closed when inspected after 48 hours. If the wound is clean, internal fixation may then be performed.

If an external fixator is used, we place two pins above and two below the wound.

Codes

GA/LA	GA
Blood	4 units
Antibiotics	Yes
Time	1 hour
Drains	0
Plaster	Yes, if not on traction
Postoperative radiograph	AP and lateral tibia
Stay	10 days

| Follow-up | 1 week |
| Off work | 3 months |

Operative requirements
- Complete external fixator and pins.
- Radiolucent operating table.
- Image intensifier and radiographer.

Postoperative care

Management
Elevate the leg on a Braun frame.

Beware compartment syndrome. If the patient has increasing pain unrelieved by splitting the dressings down to the skin, call a more senior person – do not just give stronger analgesics. Remember that fractures that have been reduced should not hurt much!

Continue antibiotic cover for at least 48 hours.

Measure the haemoglobin on the first postoperative day.

Prepare the patient to return to theatre after 48 hours, for inspection and further debridement if the wound is still dirty, or wound closure and application of a plaster cast or internal fixation if the wound is clean.

Complications
- Infection.
- Compartment syndrome.
- Deep vein thrombosis.
- Fat embolism.
- Loss of position.
- Malunion.
- Non-union.

Operation: intramedullary nail for fractured shaft of tibia

The nail is usually inserted 'closed'. That is to say that the fracture itself is not opened and the nail is passed across the fracture under radiological control.

With the patient on the orthopaedic traction table, traction is applied via a calcaneal Steinmann pin and the fracture is reduced. We

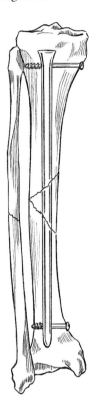

make a straight incision over the patella tendon. The approach is either just to one side or through the patella tendon. The tibial shaft is opened so that a guide wire is passed down the medullary cavity, across the fracture. Reamers are then passed over the guide wire to enlarge the medullary cavity. The nail is then passed over the guide wire.

The fracture is fixed with an interlocking nail. These have cross screws that go through both the bone and the nail, and can be inserted proximally, or distally, or both. The use of these locking screws depends on the level of the fracture in relation to the isthmus. The isthmus is the narrow mid-portion of the tibia. A fracture proximal to the isthmus needs to be locked proximally as the nail will only have a good grip in the distal fragment. A fracture distal to the isthmus needs to be locked distally as the nail will only have a good grip in the proximal fragment. If the fracture is at the isthmus or is comminuted, the nail may require locking at both ends.

Codes

GA/LA	GA
Blood	2 units
Antibiotics	Yes
Time	1.5 hours
Drains	Yes
Plaster	0
Postoperative radiograph	AP and lateral tibia
Stay	10 days
Follow-up	2 weeks
Off work	6–12 weeks

Operative requirements

- Image intensifier and radiographer.
- Orthopaedic traction table.
- A calcaneal traction pin is required, if not already *in situ*.

Postoperative care

Management

Elevate the leg on a Braun frame immediately postoperatively, prior to mobilization of the patient.

Beware compartment syndrome. If the patient has increasing pain, split the dressings down to the skin. If this does not relieve the pain, do not just give stronger analgesics, but call a senior person. Remember that reduced fractures should not hurt much!

When comfortable, the patient is mobilized either non weight-bearing or weight-bearing, depending on the stability of the fracture fixation.

Complications

- Infection.
- Compartment syndrome.
- Deep vein thrombosis.
- Fat embolism.
- Loss of position.
- Non-union.

Operation: removal of tibial intramedullary nail

The end of the nail has to be found through the original incision and exposed clearly enough for the extraction device for that particular nail to be inserted. If the end of the nail is very deep, considerable excavation of the upper end of the tibia may be required. In addition, considerable force can sometimes be needed to extract the nail. It is said that no surgeon looks good taking out metalwork!

Codes

GA/LA	GA
Blood	Group and save
Antibiotics	0
Time	30–90 minutes
Drains	Yes
Plaster	0
Postoperative radiograph	AP and lateral tibia
Stay	Day case
Follow-up	10 days
Off work	2 weeks

Operative requirements

To ensure that the correct instruments are available, theatres must know exactly what kind of nail is to be removed (Küntscher, Grosse-Kempf, AO, Richards, etc.), and if there are locking screws to be removed. If in doubt, look at the previous operating note.

High-thigh tourniquet.

Postoperative care

Management

The patient can mobilize immediately.

Complications

- Refracture during nail removal.
- Fracture not truly united.
- Infection.
- Compartment syndrome.
- Refracture postoperatively.

76 Displaced fracture of the ankle

The condition

After fractures of the hip in the elderly, ankle fractures are the most common fractures requiring inpatient care. There are several classifications, none of which are universally accepted.

When assessing an ankle fracture, you must consider whether there is injury to the malleoli, or to the medial and lateral ligaments or to the interosseous membrane. You must pay attention to the soft tissues, as their condition may determine the initial or even the definitive management of an ankle fracture. For example, an ankle that would have otherwise been internally fixed, may have to be treated in traction or with an external fixator if there is massive soft tissue swelling and fracture blisters.

Making the diagnosis

The patient

The patient may be of any age. In the young, prior to closure of the epiphyses, always remember that the ligaments are stronger than the epiphyses. In other words, children rarely have a ligamentous sprain. It is more likely that they have an epiphyseal injury and therefore must be X-rayed. In the elderly with osteoporotic bones, much less force is required to produce extremely comminuted fractures than in a young adult.

The history

Try to establish the exact mechanism of injury. Do not omit to ask where exactly the patient has pain. Always ask about pain along the whole length of the fibula.

Find out when the injury occurred. Ideally fractures should be fixed within 6 hours of the event. After that time, soft tissue swelling may delay surgery until the swelling has subsided. This may take 6 days or more.

On examination

Examine for fibula neck tenderness, especially if the patient has a medial injury but no obvious injury to the lateral side of the ankle. Palpate both sides of the ankle joint. Pain over the medial side without a medial malleolar fracture implies that there is a medial ligament injury.

Radiographs

The minimum requirement is an AP and lateral view of the ankle.

You have to see if the talus is displaced within the mortise. If there is any doubt as to whether or not there is talar shift, ask for a mortise view (45° internally rotated). Remember, that the talus is narrower posteriorly than anteriorly. This means that an AP radiograph taken with the foot in plantar flexion, may appear to have a widened gap medially. Look at the lateral view to see if the foot was indeed plantarflexed when the radiographs were taken. If necessary apply a back-slab with the foot at 90° and repeat the radiographs. The talus may now fill the mortise and 'cure' the apparent talar shift.

If there is talar shift and only a medial malleolar fracture, then the interosseous membrane must be disrupted and the fibula fractured more proximally. The fibula fracture may be as high as the fibula neck.

Preoperative management

Preparation for surgery

If the ankle is obviously dislocated – reduce it! Do not wait to get radiographs. The skin is at risk when the ankle is dislocated and prompt action can prevent a simple closed injury becoming open due to skin necrosis. Give the patient an analgesic such as entonox and/or intravenous pethidine, and then simply correct the deformity. They will be far more comfortable once the dislocation has been reduced.

Immobilize all fractures in a back-slab, even if it is only a few hours before the patient will be operated upon.

Treatment

An undisplaced stable fracture of the ankle is immobilized in a plaster cast for 6 weeks. Check radiographs are taken after 1 and 2 weeks to ensure that the position has not changed.

If the fracture is displaced, it may be possible to manipulate the fracture into an acceptable position and then immobilize the ankle in a cast.

If the fracture cannot be manipulated into a satisfactory position or if the configuration is inherently unstable, open reduction and internal fixation is necessary. Since these fractures are intra-articular in a weight bearing joint, the aim is to achieve a perfect reduction.

A very displaced fracture that needs open reduction and internal fixation may be too swollen for immediate surgery. The patient's ankle is placed in a back-slab and elevated until the soft tissue swelling diminishes.

Operation: manipulation under anaesthetic (MUA) of fractured ankle

The ankle is manipulated into as near an anatomical position as can be achieved and the position checked with either the image intensifier or plain films. Depending on the swelling around the ankle, apply either a well-padded back-slab or a full below-knee cast and splint it immediately.

Codes

GA/LA	GA
Blood	0
Antibiotics	0
Time	30 minutes
Drains	0
Plaster	Below knee
DVT prophylaxis	Yes
Postoperative radiograph	AP and lateral ankle
Stay	4 days or until internally fixed
Follow-up	1 week, X-ray on arrival
Off work	6 weeks

Operative requirements
Image intensifier and radiographer.

Postoperative care

Management

Elevate the patient's leg on pillows or a Braun frame until the patient is able to get up.

If the reduction is acceptable and no further surgery is anticipated, the patient can be mobilized non weight-bearing with crutches.

The plaster can usually be completed prior to discharge.

The ankle is kept in a cast for 6 weeks.

Complications

- Fracture blisters.
- Loss of reduction of the fracture.
- Deep vein thrombosis.
- Compartment syndrome.

Operation: open reduction and internal fixation (ORIF) of a fractured ankle

The medial malleolus is usually held by two parallel screws which are inserted near the tip of the malleolus and pass perpendicular to the fracture line.

The lateral malleolus is usually fixed using interfragmentary screws plus a plate. The exact arrangement depends on the configuration of the fracture.

Codes

GA/LA	GA
Blood	0
Antibiotics	Yes
Time	1–2 hours
Drains	Yes
Plaster	Below-knee back-slab
DVT prophylaxis	Yes
Postoperative radiograph	AP and lateral ankle
Stay	3 days
Follow-up	10 days
Off work	6 weeks

Operative requirements

- Small fragment AO set.
- Radiolucent operating table.
- Plain films or image intensifier to check on the fixation.
- A tourniquet is commonly used, but is in fact unnecessary if the leg is elevated in the Trendelenburg position during surgery.

Postoperative care

Management

Elevate the patient's leg while the patient is in bed. Remove the drains after 24 hours.

There are two schools of thought about postoperative care of ankle fractures. Some surgeons simply leave the ankle in a plaster cast for 6 weeks. Others insist on immediate active movement postoperatively. Active ankle movement out of the back-slab is commenced after 24 hours. When the patient can actively bring the ankle to 90°, a full below-knee plaster is applied. This early mobilization will mean that movement will be much better when the plaster comes off. However the long-term results are very similar between patients who are not mobilized prior to going into a cast and those that are.

The ankle remains in a cast for a total of 6 weeks. Two weeks non weight-bearing and then weight-bearing for 4 weeks.

Complications

- Wound breakdown.
- Wound infection.
- Compartment syndrome.
- Deep vein thrombosis.
- Loss of position if the fixation is inadequate or the bone is very osteoporotic.
- Late osteoarthritis.

Operation: removal of internal fixation from the ankle

The screws and plates are removed through the original incisions. This is done in the young (less than 40 years), with a healed fracture, at least 18 months following internal fixation.

Codes

GA/LA	GA
Blood	0
Antibiotics	0
Time	1 hour
Drains	Optional
Plaster	0
Postoperative radiograph	0
Stay	Day case
Follow-up	10 days
Off work	2 weeks

Operative requirements

- Tourniquet.
- Inform theatres as to what kind of metalwork is to be removed – whether small or large fragment AO. If in doubt look at the old operating note.

Postoperative care

Management

The patient may be fully weight-bearing immediately. They should avoid high risk activities, such as contact sports, for about 6 weeks to allow the holes in the bones to heal.

Complications

- Poor wound healing.
- Fracture not truly united.
- Refracture postoperatively.

CHAPTER 77

Arthritis of the ankle joint

The condition

Osteoarthritis of the ankle is unusual. It may occur secondary to a fracture of the ankle or talus. Alternatively, it may be secondary to osteochondritis of the talus.

The ankle is commonly affected in rheumatoid arthritis.

Following a displaced ankle fracture, arthritis is unlikely to develop if the joint has been anatomically reconstructed. However, if the joint is not returned to a congruent state, secondary degeneration is very likely and will be evident on the radiographs 18 months following the injury.

Making the diagnosis

The history

The most important symptom to assess is pain:

- Assess the severity and the frequency of the pain.
- What painkillers does the patient take to relieve the pain and how often?
- How far can the patient walk before they have to stop because of pain?
- Does the patient walk with a stick?
- Does pain from the ankle wake the patient at night?

On examination

Watch the patient walk. Do they limp? Do they use a stick?

Look for, and document, the position of any scars.

Examine the patient standing from behind and compare the alignment of the heels. Is the heel in valgus or varus?

Examine and compare the movements in both ankles. Be sure to separate the movement at the ankle joint itself, from movement at the subtalar joint and the midtarsal joint. The movements of the ankle are best expressed as degrees of dorsi- and plantar flexion, whereas the subtalar and midfoot are best expressed as percentages of the normal.

Feel for foot pulses. Examine sensation in the toes.

Radiographs
AP and lateral views of the ankle are usually adequate.

Treatment

Indications for surgery
A painful ankle that is not improving, at least 18 months following the original injury.

Operation: arthrodesis of the ankle

This can be performed in a variety of ways. The ankle can either be approached medially, by detaching the medial malleolus, or anteriorly via a transverse or longitudinal incision or posteriorly after dividing the Achilles tendon. The articular surfaces of the tibia and the talus are denuded of cartilage and the surfaces made parallel.

Iliac crest bone graft is usually used to fill the gap between the bone surfaces.

The arthrodesis can be held with external compression clamps or with plates and screws.

Codes
GA/LA	GA
Blood	Group and save
Antibiotics	Yes
Time	1.5 hours
Drains	Yes
Plaster	Yes, below knee
DVT Prophylaxis	Yes
Postoperative radiograph	AP and lateral ankle
Stay	5 days
Follow-up	6 weeks
Off work	2–3 months

Operative requirements
- Thigh tourniquet.
- Compression clamp or AO plating set.
- Include on the consent and the operating list, the possibility of taking iliac crest bone graft.

Postoperative care

Management
Elevate the leg immediately postoperatively. Watch for compartment syndrome and wound problems.

   Once the wound is stable, a below-knee plaster cast is applied and the patient mobilized non weight-bearing. After 6 weeks, the cast is changed to a weight-bearing cast. This is kept on until the ankle is clinically and radiologically united. This may take up to 14 weeks.

Complications
- Neuro-vascular damage.
- Poor position of fusion.
- Failure of fusion.

78

Arthritis of the subtalar and midtarsal joints

The condition

The subtalar and the talo-navicular and the calcaneocuboid joints can be affected by rheumatoid arthritis. More commonly, previous fracture of the talus or the calcaneum can lead to secondary osteoarthritis of subtalar joint.

Making the diagnosis

The history

The most important symptom to assess is pain:

- Assess the severity and the frequency of the patient's pain.
- What medication does the patient take and how much?
- How far can the patient walk before stopping because of pain?
- Does the patient use a walking stick?
- Does the pain wake the patient at night?

On examination

Watch the patient walk. Does he limp? Does he use a stick?

Look for and document the position of any scars.

Examine the patient standing from behind and compare the alignment of the heels. Is the heel in valgus or varus?

Look for callosities from weight bearing in an abnormal fashion.

Compare the range of movements in both ankles and feet. Be sure to separate the movements that occur in the ankle joint itself, from movement at the subtalar joint and the midtarsal joint. The movements of the ankle are best expressed as degrees of dorsi- and plantar flexion, whereas the subtalar and mid-foot are best expressed as percentages of the normal. Also note which movements the patient finds painful.

Feel for the foot pulses. Check that sensation in the toes is normal.

Radiographs
Request AP and lateral views of the ankle and the foot.

Treatment

Indications for surgery

Arthrodesis of the tarsal joints is indicated either to stabilize and realign a paralysed foot or in the treatment of severe arthritis affecting the tarsal joints.

Fracture of the calcaneum can result in arthritis in the subtalar joint. If this is the only joint affected, we only arthrodese the subtalar fusion.

Operation: triple arthrodesis of the tarsal joints (combined subtalar and midtarsal arthrodesis)

The joints that are fused are the subtalar joint, the calcaneo-cuboid joint and the talo-navicular joint. This is done through a laterally based incision. The articular surface of the joints is removed and the bone surfaces apposed. If necessary, a wedge of bone is removed to correct a fixed deformity. The bones are usually held together using bone staples.

Codes

GA/LA	GA
Blood	Group and save
Antibiotics	Yes
Time	1 hour
Drains	0
Plaster	Yes, below knee
DVT prophylaxis	Yes
Postoperative radiograph	Whole foot
Stay	5 days
Follow-up	6 weeks
Off work	2–3 months

Operative requirements

- Tourniquet.
- Bone staples.

Postoperative care

Management

Elevate the leg postoperatively until the patient is mobilized. The patient remains non weight-bearing between crutches for 5 weeks. After that time the patient is kept in a walking cast until there is clinical and radiological union.

Complications

- Compartment syndrome.
- Poor position of fusion.
- Failure of fusion.
- Continued pain despite radiological fusion.

79

Rupture of the Achilles' tendon

The condition

Rupture of the Achilles' tendon (also known as the tendo Achillis – note the spelling) is common in the fourth and fifth decades. The tendon ruptures due to degeneration of the tendon combined with a sudden force passing along the tendon.

Making the diagnosis

The patient
Commonly, the patient is a man in his early forties who has been playing a sport such as squash or football.

The history
The patient will often describe the feeling that he had been struck on the back of the heel by their opponent's racquet – when he had not. He complains of severe pain just above the heel.

On examination
With a complete rupture of the Achilles' tendon, there is bruising around the back of the heel and tenderness. There is usually a palpable gap between the ends of the ruptured tendon. The patient will not be able to stand on tiptoe.

Simmond's test is the definitive test for a ruptured Achilles' tendon. It is best performed with the patient kneeling on a chair. Squeeze the patient's calves one at a time. On the normal leg, squeezing the calf makes the ankle plantar flex. If there is a complete rupture of the Achilles' tendon, squeezing the calf does not produce plantar flexion of the ankle.

Radiographs

A lateral view of the calcaneum should be taken to exclude avulsion of the tendon complete with a bony fragment. This is extremely rare. (If a bony fragment has been avulsed, it needs to be reduced and fixed in place.)

If there is any doubt as to the diagnosis, an ultrasound will demonstrate a tear in the tendon. Some surgeons like an ultrasound to assess if passive full dorsiflexion of the ankle brings the two ends of the ruptured tendon together. If it does, then they are happy to treat the patient conservatively in a cast.

Treatment

A complete tear that is seen within a few hours of the injury is treated conservatively in a plaster. The cast is applied with the ankle maximally dorsiflexed. Some surgeons insist on an above-knee cast. Others feel that a below-knee cast is satisfactory. The cast is kept on for 8 weeks.

If the patient is seen more than 24 hours after the injury most surgeons agree that surgery is required.

Indications for surgery

A complete rupture of the tendo Achillis.

Operation: repair of ruptured Achilles' tendon

We make a posterior longitudinal incision just lateral to the midline. The tendon ends are brought together and sutured. Suturing the ruptured tendon is difficult because the ends of the tendon are very ragged. Nevertheless, as long as the ends are apposed the tendon should heal. Postoperatively, the repair is protected by placing the leg in a cast with the ankle plantar flexed.

Codes

GA/LA	GA
Blood	0
Antibiotics	Optional
Time	1 hour
Drains	0
Plaster	Below knee with the ankle plantar flexed

DVT prophylaxis	Yes
Postoperative radiograph	0
Stay	4 days
Follow-up	2 weeks
Off work	8 weeks

Operative requirements

- Tourniquet.
- The operation is performed with the patient prone. You should warn the anaesthetist about this so that he inserts a guarded endotracheal tube.

Postoperative care

Management

When comfortable, the patient is mobilized non weight-bearing.

The exact regime of outpatient care should be clearly stated by the surgeon in the operation notes as there are several alternatives. A safe regime is:

(a) a below-knee cast with the ankle fully plantar flexed for 4 weeks;

(b) the cast is then changed to one with the ankle only partly plantar flexed, for 4 more weeks;

(c) once out of plaster, the patient should wear a shoe raise for 2 weeks.

The patient should only be allowed to play sport when he is able to stand on tiptoe.

Complications

- Poor wound healing.
- Wound infection.
- Re-rupture (approximately 10%).
- Rupture of the other Achilles' tendon.

CHAPTER

80

Fracture of the calcaneum

The condition

The calcaneum is also referred to as the os calcis.

A calcaneal fracture commonly results from a fall where the patient lands on his feet. It is a common fracture. The long-term result following a displaced fracture is often poor.

Making the diagnosis

The history

The patient will have fallen from a considerable height. He complains of a painful heel and foot. He may have tried to weight bear but found it too painful. It is important to ask the patient if he has pain anywhere else, especially in the back.

On examination

Examine the foot and ankle with care. The common sign of a calcaneal injury is bruising on the instep of the foot that is like a thumb print.

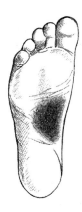

This is because the attachment of the plantar fascia limits the spread of the haematoma. Compare the width of the patient's heels. Note if the injured side is wider than the uninjured side.

Palpate the patient's spine. Tenderness in the thoraco-lumbar junction may be due to a vertebral crush fracture.

Radiographs

Order views of the calcaneum and the lumbar spine. The hind foot views should include a lateral, two obliques and an axial view.

If surgery is contemplated, you will need to order a CT scan of the hind foot taken in the coronal plane.

Preoperative management

Common associated injuries

Crush fracture of the first lumbar vertebra.

Treatment

Most patients with a calcaneal fracture need to be admitted as they usually develop considerable swelling.

Place the leg in a below-knee back-slab with the ankle at 90°. Elevate the leg on a Braun frame and instruct the nursing staff to apply regular ice packs.

The majority of calcaneal fractures are treated conservatively. Once the swelling has subsided, a below-knee plaster cast is applied and the patient is mobilized non weight-bearing with crutches.

Indications for surgery

There is considerable debate about the value of surgery. Due to the soft cancellous nature of the bone, manipulation of the fragments and insertion of screws is exceedingly difficult. However, a calcaneal fracture with depression of the subtalar joint, that is not comminuted, is suitable for elevation of the joint surface and internal fixation.

Operation: open reduction and elevation of calcaneal fracture

The fracture is exposed through a lateral incision. The aim is to elevate the articular surface of the subtalar joint and then to pack in bone graft to help keep the joint surface elevated.

Codes

GA/LA	GA
Blood	Group and save
Antibiotics	Yes
Time	1 hour
Drains	0
Plaster	Below knee
DVT prophylaxis	Yes
Postoperative radiograph	Calcaneal views
Stay	1 week
Follow-up	4 weeks
Off work	2–3 months

Operative requirements

■ Tourniquet.

■ Obtain consent for, and include on the theatre list, the possibility of taking iliac crest bone graft.

Postoperative care

Management

Keep the leg elevated on pillows or a Braun frame until the patient is comfortable enough to mobilize. Then mobilize the patient non weight-bearing between crutches.

Complications

■ Wound infection.

■ Subtalar arthritis.

CHAPTER 8

Congenital talipes equino-varus (club foot)

The condition

This is a common congenital foot deformity (about 1–2 per 1,000 live births). It is more common in males and is bilateral in one third of cases. Talipes means club foot. The deformity is a combination of:

1. The talus pointing down and out – bringing the hind foot into *equinus*.

2. The navicular and the fore foot being shifted medially with additional supination – giving the *varus* deformity of the forefoot.

Making the diagnosis

The patient
The deformity is usually detected at birth.

On examination
Gently take the baby's foot and bring it up and out. If the foot can be brought into a normal position the deformity is referred to as 'correctable'.

You must check for the associated conditions of spina bifida and arthrogryposis.

Radiographs
Radiographs in the newborn are not very helpful. Later, when the bones begin to ossify, the relationship of the talus to the calcaneum is measured on the AP and lateral views of the foot.

Treatment

Treatment must begin on presentation, with strapping of the baby's foot in as near a corrected position as possible. The strapping is applied without an anaesthetic and is replaced weekly. If at 6 weeks a full correction has not been achieved, operative correction is necessary.

Operation: postero-medial release for club foot

The aim is to divide or elongate any structures on the medial and posterior part of the foot that are preventing the foot from assuming a normal position. This may include elongation of the tendo Achillis, the tendons of tibialis posterior, flexor digitorum longus and flexor hallucis longus, and division of the capsule of the subtalar, talo-navicular and calcaneo-cuboid joints.

At the end of the operation, it should be possible to bring the foot into a normal attitude.

Codes

GA/LA	GA
Blood	0
Antibiotics	0
Time	1.5 hours
Drains	0
Plaster	Above knee, for 6 weeks
Postoperative radiograph	0
Stay	4 days
Follow-up	2 weeks

Operative requirement
Paediatric tourniquet.

Postoperative care

Management
After 2 weeks, when the wound is healed, the definitive plaster is applied with the foot in the fully corrected position. The foot is kept in a plaster cast for 6 weeks.

Following removal of the plaster, the child wears special splints (Denis Browne boots) to prevent the deformity recurring. Splintage usually continues until the age of one.

Complications

- Injury to the posterior tibial neuro-vascular bundle.
- Wound breakdown.
- Incomplete correction of the deformity.
- Recurrence of the deformity.

Clawed toes

The condition

In children, clawing of the toes may be idiopathic or secondary to a neurological disorder. In an adult, the deformity may occur in an otherwise normal foot, or with a hallux valgus, or as a result of rheumatoid arthritis.

Making the diagnosis

The history

The patient complains of pain under the ball of the foot and callosities. The prominent proximal interphalangeal joints may also be sore. The patient complains that he cannot find a comfortable pair of shoes to wear.

On examination

In claw toes, the metatarsal phalangeal joints are hyperextended and are often subluxated or dislocated. The proximal and the distal interphalangeal joints are both held flexed.

Look for callosities underneath the metatarsal heads and on the dorsum of the prominent proximal interphalangeal joint of the toes.

Check the neuro-vascular status of the foot, in particular the presence or absence of foot pulses.

Examine the back of a child who has claw toes. A dimple or hairy patch in the lower lumbar region may indicate spina bifida occulta.

Radiographs

Order radiographs of the foot to exclude any other cause for pain. Look to see if any of the metatarsophalangeal joints are dislocated.

Treatment

Indications for surgery

If the toes can be passively straightened, a dynamic correction can be performed to realign the toes (Girdlestone's procedure).

If the deformity is fixed (cannot be passively corrected) but the metatarsophalangeal joints are not dislocated, (Helal's) metatarsal osteotomies are performed.

For a severe fixed deformity, where the metatarsophalangeal joints are dislocated, a forefoot arthroplasty is performed.

Operation: flexor to extensor transfer of toes (Girdlestone's procedure)

The long flexor of each toe is transferred into the extensor expansion over the dorsum of the proximal phalanx. This is done through lateral incisions on the second, third and fourth toes.

Codes

GA/LA	GA
Blood	0
Antibiotics	0
Time	45 minutes
Drains	0
Plaster	0
DVT prophylaxis	Yes
Postoperative radiograph	0
Stay	2 days
Follow-up	2 weeks
Off work	6 weeks

Operative requirement
Tourniquet.

Postoperative care

Management
The toes may be held straight by strips of plaster of Paris on the dorsum of the toe. If used, these are kept on for 2 weeks.

The patient is mobilized fully weight-bearing, as soon as the pain allows.

Complication
Inadequate correction.

Operation: dorsal displacement osteotomy of the metatarsal shafts (Helal's osteotomies)

A longitudinal dorsal incision is made between adjacent metatarsals so that the two can be operated upon through a single incision. The metatarsal necks are divided obliquely so that the metatarsal heads slide proximally and dorsally. No internal fixation is required. As a result the metatarsal heads are less prominent and the shortening of the metatarsal reduces the clawing of the toe.

Codes

GA/LA	GA
Blood	0
Antibiotics	0
Time	30 minutes
Drains	0
Plaster	0
Postoperative radiograph	AP and lateral forefoot
Stay	2–3 nights
Follow-up	2 weeks
Off work	6–10 weeks

Operative requirement
Tourniquet.

Postoperative care

Management
The patient mobilizes walking on their heel as their pains allows.

When the pain subsides, the patient should be encouraged to weight bear on the front of the foot, otherwise the metatarsal heads may fall back into their original position.

Complications
- Division of both neuro-vascular bundles to a toe.
- Poor position of osteotomy.
- Non-union.

Operation: forefoot arthroplasty (Kates-Kessel or Fowler's procedure)

In a simple (Kates-Kessel) forefoot arthroplasty, only the distal ends of the metatarsals are excised. This removes the prominent metatarsal heads and the resultant shortening of the toes relaxes the clawing. This procedure is performed through three separate longitudinal dorsal incisions.

In a Fowler's procedure, the bases of the proximal phalanges as well as the distal ends of the metatarsals are excised – in other words it is an excision arthroplasty of the metatarsophalangeal joints. In addition, an ellipse of plantar skin can be excised to draw back the anteriorly displaced pad of weight-bearing skin into its correct position.

Since both procedures shorten the foot, they should be performed on both feet and not on a single foot.

Codes
GA/LA	GA
Blood	0
Antibiotics	Optional
Time	1 hour
Drains	0
DVT prophylaxis	Yes
Plaster	0
Postoperative radiograph	AP feet
Stay	2 weeks
Follow-up	6 weeks
Off work	3 months

Operative requirements
- Tourniquet.
- Powered saw.

Postoperative care

Management

Elevate the feet and keep the patient non weight-bearing until the wounds have healed.

Once the wounds are stable, the patient can mobilize full weight-bearing as the pain allows.

Complications

- Injury to the neuro-vascular supply to a digit, leading to loss of a toe. This is a greater risk with the Fowler's procedure.
- Wound infection.
- Persistent pain.
- Slow recovery.

Hammer toe

The condition

This common condition is of unknown aetiology and commonly affects the second toe.

Making the diagnosis

The history

The patient complains of soreness over the proximal interphalangeal joint of the toe that is unrelieved by proprietary pads and plasters.

On examination

A hammer toe is a fixed deformity (cannot be passively corrected) and is equivalent to a boutonnière deformity in the finger – the metatarso-phalangeal and distal interphalangeal joints are hyperextended while the proximal interphalangeal joint is flexed and thus prominent.

Treatment

Indication for surgery

Painful hammer toe.

Operation: fusion of the proximal interphalangeal joint for hammer toe

We make an elliptical incision over the dorsum of the proximal inter-phalangeal joint. We divide the extensor tendon. We then cut the ends off the proximal phalanx and the middle phalanx so excising the joint. Some surgeons hold the toe straight with a K-wire that is brought out through the end of the toe. Others just sew the extensor tendon and the skin, and let the toe fuse with the toe slightly flexed. If used, the wire is removed in the clinic after 6 weeks.

Codes

GA/LA	GA
Blood	0
Antibiotics	0
Time	30 minutes
Drains	0
Plaster	0
Postoperative radiograph	0
Stay	Day case
Follow-up	10 days
Off work	6 weeks

Operative requirements

- Tourniquet.
- K-wire set and driver.

Postoperative care

Management

Check to see that the toe becomes pink once the tourniquet has been deflated. If the toe remains dusky, this may be due either to the vessels being stretched and/or the dressings being too tight. Push the end of the toe down the K-wire to reduce possible stretching of the vessels. Release the dressings around the toe. The toe should become pink. If the toe still looks dusky call the surgeon who performed the surgery.

If only one toe is fused, the patient is able to mobilize with little discomfort. If multiple toes are fused, the patient may be able to be discharged after 1 or 2 nights. He should rest at home with his legs elevated until the foot is comfortable enough to walk upon.

The wire is removed after 6 weeks, in the clinic.

Complications

- Non-union of fusion.
- Division of both neuro-vascular bundles to a digit.

84

CHAPTER

Hallux valgus

The condition

Hallux valgus is the deformity of the big toe where the toe is angled away from the midline of the body and thus is in valgus. The metatarsal of the big toe may be displaced towards the other foot and may be in varus. The condition may be familial or it may be acquired.

A bunion is the inflamed bursa that lies on the side of the metatarsophalangeal joint.

Making the diagnosis

The patient
The patient is usually a middle-aged female, although if the problem is congenital, the patient may present in the second or third decade.

The history
The main complaints are pain over the prominence on the medial side of the metatarsophalangeal joint and a widened foot that makes buying shoes difficult. If there is an adventitial bursa, this may become inflamed and give episodes of pain. There may be a family history of the condition.

On examination
The metatarsophalangeal joint is prominent and there may be a painful bursa over the joint. The great toe may be so angulated that it presses on or under the second toe.

Examine the great toe and see if it can be brought into a normal position.

Examine the range of flexion and extension of the metatarsophalangeal joint. If the joint is stiff, the pain may be due to osteoarthritis rather than hallux valgus.

329

Always check on the neurovascular status of the foot, especially if the patient is a diabetic.

Radiographs

Order standing AP and lateral radiographs of the foot. They will show the degree of deformity when the patient is weight-bearing. On the AP, you should measure the angle formed by the metatarsal and the proximal phalanx. Look at the metatarsophalangeal joint to see if there is degenerative change.

Treatment

Indications for surgery

Deformity itself is not a reason to operate, however unsightly. Surgery is only indicated if the patient has persistent pain.

There are many different operations for hallux valgus:

If the patient is under 70 years, without arthritis of the metatarsophalangeal joint, most surgeons perform some type of metatarsal osteotomy. The choice of osteotomy partly depends on the degree of valgus:

(a) if the valgus at the metatarsophalangeal joint is less than 30° on the standing radiograph and is fully correctable on examination, a displacement osteotomy is adequate, e.g. chevron osteotomy;

(b) if the valgus is greater than 30°, the metatarsal osteotomy should shorten the metatarsal a little to give the additional correction, e.g. Hohmann's or Mitchell's osteotomies.

In a patient over 70 years, the simplest operation is to remove the proximal third of the proximal phalanx (Keller's excision arthroplasty) and the bony prominence.

Operation: chevron metatarsal osteotomy

We make a dorso-medial incision centred over the first metatarsophalangeal joint. We remove the bony prominence on the medial side of the metatarsal head. An osteotomy is performed that displaces the metatarsal shaft laterally (towards the second toe) without any angulation. Because of its design (like the letter V on its side with the tip pointing distally), the osteotomy is very stable.

Codes

GA/LA	GA
Blood	0
Antibiotics	Optional
Time	30 minutes
Drains	0
Plaster	Plaster slipper
Postoperative radiograph	AP and lateral great toe
Stay	Overnight
Follow-up	3 weeks
Off work	6 weeks

Operative requirements
- Tourniquet.
- Fine power saw.

Postoperative care

Management
The patient keeps his foot elevated until comfortable enough to mobilize. The patient can then walk heel-bearing.

After 3 weeks the plaster slipper is changed and the patient can weight bear on the whole foot.

Complications
- Wound infection.
- Loss of position of osteotomy.
- Non-union.
- Persistent pain.
- Avascular necrosis of the metatarsal head.

Operation: Mitchell's metatarsal osteotomy

We make a dorso-medial incision, centred over the first metatarso-phalangeal joint. We remove the bony prominence on the medial side of the metatarsal head. We then make two cuts across the neck of the metatarsal. The more proximal goes all the way across the bone. The more distal cut is incomplete in order to leave a lateral spike on the distal fragment that will keep the head displaced laterally. The distal fragment is displaced laterally and the two fragments impacted together. The medial capsule is reefed to help hold the toe straight. A K-wire or a staple can be used to hold the osteotomy.

Codes

GA/LA	GA
Blood	0
Antibiotics	0
Time	30 minutes
Drains	0
Plaster	Yes, if K-wire or staple are not used
Postoperative radiograph	AP and lateral great toe
Stay	Overnight
Follow-up	2 weeks
Off work	6 weeks

Operative requirements

- Tourniquet.
- Power saw, drill and K-wire (if required).
- Staple gun (if required).

Postoperative care

Management

Elevate the leg initially.

The patient mobilizes bearing weight on his heel. The sutures are removed after 2 weeks. The K-wire is removed as a day-case under a brief GA after 6 weeks.

If no internal fixation is used, the plaster is changed after 2 weeks to a plaster slipper in which the patient remains for 4 more weeks.

Complications

- Non-union.
- Poor position of fusion.
- Metatarsalgia under the metatarsal heads of the second to fifth toes.

Operation: Keller's excision arthroplasty

The joint is exposed through a dorso-medial incision. The bony prominence under the bunion and the proximal half of the proximal phalanx are removed. When it has healed, the great toe is short and is a little floppy.

Codes

GA/LA	GA
Blood	0
Antibiotics	0
Time	30 minutes
Drains	0
Plaster	0
Postoperative radiograph	(Optional) AP and lateral toe
Stay	Overnight
Follow-up	2 weeks
Off work	6 weeks

Operative requirement
Tourniquet.

Postoperative care

Management
- Elevate the leg initially.
- Allow the patient to weight bear as the pain allows.

Complication
Too generous a resection of the proximal phalanx.

Arthritis of the great toe MTP joint

The condition

Hallux rigidus is essentially arthritis of the great toe MTP joint. It may develop from an injury that occurred many years previously, but the cause is often not known.

Making the diagnosis

The patient
The patient is usually in their middle age.

The history
The patient complains of pain in the MTP joint that is made worse on walking. Women may note that they have difficulty wearing as high a heel as they wore previously.

On examination
Examine the range of dorsiflexion and plantar flexion at the MTP joint. Note the range of movement, whether movement causes pain and if there is crepitus. Compare both sides.

Radiographs
Ask for AP standing, and lateral views of the foot.

Treatment

Indications for surgery
Surgery is indicated if the pain interferes with daily life and anti-inflammatory medication has not helped.

Operation: arthrodesis of the first MTP joint

We make an incision along the dorso-medial aspect of the joint. We denude the joint surfaces of any remaining articular cartilage. The surfaces are trimmed so that there is good bone to bone contact in the desired position. The bones are held in place with a bone staple or a screw.

Codes

GA/LA	GA
Blood	0
Antibiotics	Yes
Time	1 hour
Drains	0
Plaster	Forefoot
Postoperative radiograph	AP and lateral foot
Stay	1 night
Follow-up	10 days
Off work	4 weeks minimum

Operative requirements

- Tourniquet.
- Bone staple or small fragment screw set.

Postoperative care

Management

- Elevate the leg initially.
- The patient takes weight on the heel of the operated foot while in a plaster.

Complications

- Infection.
- Failure of the bone to fuse.
- Fusion in an unsatisfactory position (e.g. too dorsiflexed).

86

Morton's neuroma

The condition

Morton's neuroma is the name used to describe swelling of a digital nerve in the foot. The neuroma typically occurs just before or just after the common digital nerve divides into two. The neuroma causes metatarsalgia – pain under the metatarsal head.

Making the diagnosis

The patient
Although it can occur at any age, the patient is usually over the age of 40. It is more common in women.

The history
The patient complains of extreme pain under the ball of the foot when weight-bearing. She may describe the pain as feeling as if she is walking on broken glass. The patient may have noticed abnormal sensation in the toe supplied by the nerve.

On examination
Squeeze the metatarsal heads together. You may be able to elicit a palpable clunk that is accompanied by pain. Carefully palpate the ball of the foot. It is usually possible to identify one spot that is the most sensitive. Do not forget to examine sensation in the toes.

Radiographs
Obtain radiographs of the foot to exclude any bony cause for the pain. Ultrasound is a reliable method for identifying a neuroma. The accuracy is dependent on the skill of the ultrasonographer.

Preoperative management

Preparation for surgery

Describe the operation exactly on the consent form. If the surgeon always excises the nerve, the patient must consent to this, e.g. *excision of the digital nerve to the cleft of left 4th/5th toes.*

Clearly mark the affected cleft preoperatively on both the dorsum and plantar surfaces of the foot.

Warn the patient that the toes that are involved may be permanently numb following surgery.

Treatment

Indications for surgery

Symptoms and signs of a digital neuroma that has not responded to conservative treatment with pads, etc.

The traditional treatment is to excise the abnormal nerve. This has the disadvantage of leaving behind a cut nerve end which may go on to form a neuroma that may become symptomatic.

Some surgeons prefer to preserve the nerve. If there is an obvious cause for nerve compression such as a ganglion, the ganglion is excised. If there is no obvious cause of nerve compression the surgeon divides the intermetatarsal ligament. This allows the metatarsals to separate and give the digital nerve more room.

Operation: excision of plantar digital neuroma for Morton's metatarsalgia

The digital nerve is exposed through either a plantar or a dorsal longitudinal incision centred on the correct interspace. The common digital nerve (i.e. before it divides into two separate digital nerves) is located and is usually visibly enlarged. The nerve is excised. Due to the excision of the nerve, the toe web may be permanently numb after surgery, but pain free.

If the nerve is simply decompressed, the incision and approach are the same. The toes are not numb afterwards.

Codes

GA/LA	GA
Blood	0
Antibiotics	0
Time	30 minutes
Drains	0
Plaster	0
Postoperative radiograph	0
Stay	Day case
Follow-up	10 days
Off work	3–6 weeks

Operative requirements

- Tourniquet.
- Send the resected nerve to histology to confirm that a nerve was resected and there was a neuroma. (This is very useful should the operation not be a success!)

Postoperative care

Management

The patient may mobilize immediately. He must keep the leg elevated when not walking for the first few days.

Complications

- Wrong diagnosis, leading to persistence of symptoms.
- Tender scar.

87

Foreign body in the foot

The condition

This is remarkably common injury. The foreign body is commonly a pin or a broken needle.

Making the diagnosis

The history
The patient usually presents on the day of injury, pretty certain that they have stepped on 'something' and complaining of pain in the foot.

On examination
There may be a tiny puncture hole where the foreign body entered. If the injury occurred several days previously, look for signs of cellulitis or abscess formation.

Radiographs
Ask for radiographs of the foot in two planes, with a marker taped to the skin to indicate the entry hole. You will be surprised how far away the foreign body may be from its entry point.

If the radiographs are normal and the patient is certain that they have trodden on something, order an ultrasound. This will detect a foreign body that is radiolucent such as a wooden cocktail stick.

Treatment

Unless you can actually see the end of the pin/needle, do not attempt to remove it in casualty under local anaesthesia. It can literally be like looking for a needle in a haystack and is often difficult for the surgeon and painful for the patient.

Indications for surgery
Any foreign body in the foot that is causing pain.

Operation: removal of foreign body from the foot

This is often a trickier procedure than you might expect. With the patient prone, we locate the foreign body with the image intensifier. We put two hypodermic needles into the sole of the foot at right angles to each other, to establish the position of the object. We make a cut and then find the object by a combination of screening with the image intensifier and feeling with an artery clip.

Codes

GA/LA	GA
Blood	0
Antibiotics	Yes
Time	30 minutes–1 hour
Drains	0
Plaster	0
Postoperative radiograph	0
Stay	Day case or overnight
Follow-up	10 days
Off work	10 days

Operative requirements
- Tourniquet.
- Image intensifier and radiographer.

Postoperative care

Management
The patient may weight bear immediately, within the limit of their discomfort.

Complications
- Inability to retrieve the foreign body.
- Wound infection.

Glossary

AO. Association for Osteosynthesis. This refers to the system of fracture fixation originated by the Swiss.

AO mini-fragment set. Set of plates and screws used for fixing fractures in the hand.

AO small fragment set. Set of plates and screws used to fixing forearm and ankle fractures.

AO standard fragment set. Set of plates and screws suitable for fixing large adult bones.

Arthrodesis. Surgical fusion of a joint.

Arthroplasty. An operation that restores function to a joint. This is commonly by replacement with an artificial joint, but not always. Excision of the joint without replacement is also an arthroplasty.

Calcar. The calcar is the relatively strong medial neck of the femur above the level of the lesser trochanter.

Closed (fracture). A fracture without an associated skin defect.

Comminuted. A term used to describe a fracture when the bone is in many pieces.

Compound (fracture). A fracture associated with a skin wound. Also referred to as an open fracture.

CPM (continuous passive motion). The CPM machine is a machine containing a motor that bends and straightens the limb passively. The range and the rate of movement are adjustable.

Denham pin. A traction 'pin' that is up to 20 cm long and 5 mm in diameter. It is threaded in the middle third to prevent it sliding out of the bone.

Image intensifier. An X-ray machine that produces an instant image on a television monitor.

Kirschner wire, K-wire. A sharp stout 'pin' that may be between 10 and 20 cm long, and of various widths from 0.9 to 3 mm. It is inserted either using a hand-held chuck or with a powered K-wire driver.

Kuntscher nail, K-nail. A long steel nail, used for the intramedullary fixation of fractures.

MUA. Manipulation under anaesthesia.

ORIF. Open reduction and internal fixation (of a fracture).

Osteotomy. A general term for surgical division of a bone.

Patella, patellar. Patella is the bone itself. Patellar is the adjective that refers to the bone.

Radiculogram. The radiological study of the spinal nerve roots and their sheaths after the injection of a radiopacque contrast medium, which is water soluble.

Revision. In reference to operations, a revision is a second operation of the same nature as the first.

Steinmann pin. A traction 'pin' that is up to 20 cm long and 5 mm in diameter. It is smooth throughout (in contrast to a Denham pin).

TED. Thromboembolic deterrent (stocking).

Tomogram. A radiograph produced by tomography, where each image is of one layer of the body at any required depth.

Ulna, ulnar. Ulna is the bone itself. Ulnar is the adjective referring to the ulna (on the ulnar side ...).

Volar. A synonym for palmar or plantar.

Index

Index